AUTOPHAGY

How to Use Your Body's Natural Intelligence for
Self-Cleansing, Anti-Aging, and Rapid Weight Loss

Avery Hansen

Table of Contents

Introduction

What was your reaction when you heard the word "autophagy" for the first time? Or could this be the first time you're reading about it? It's quite a mouthful, and it sounds terribly complicated, something that only medical professionals should be familiar with. The first time I read about autophagy, the author went to a lot of trouble to help us readers understand the pronunciation, which I can understand, but I couldn't help giggling at the demonstration. It was something like *Aah - toh - fah - jee*. It was very useful, so I must give the author credit for that. My partner, however, refused to accept that this was the correct pronunciation, so we had to search a YouTube channel that pronounces words—one that he deemed "credible," of course. He listened to the robot voice several times while giving me dirty looks, but he finally caved. Only then was I triumphant.

The most fascinating thing about the word Autophagy, for me, is what it means. The word is of Greek origin, and it actually consists of two components, "auto" and "phagy." "Auto" means "self" and "phagy" means "eat," which leaves you with the concept of "self-eating" (Lindberg & Murrell, 2018). I must admit, if one is not familiar with the functions and benefits of autophagy, the idea can be kind of creepy and even gross; how can there be hype about something that sounds so unnatural, especially in the beauty industry? Well, the biggest surprise you will get when you start learning about autophagy is that it's the polar opposite of unnatural. It's unbelievable, and you would never have thought that the body had this kind of superpowers and astonishing intelligence. Let's talk about what autophagy is and why its existence was such a ground-breaking discovery.

Autophagy is not understood as only a state that the body enters, but also as an ongoing process, and it is the body's way of "spring-cleaning" itself to get rid of unwanted debris that may be irritating the body and preventing growth and healing, like inflammation. This aforementioned act of "spring-cleaning" is synonymous with the self-eating or self-cannibalizing we mentioned earlier, and this connection comes from the way the body reuses or recycles the unwanted debris for the generation and production of new cells or for cell repair. This process is identified as an evolutionary and self-preserving mechanism that helps the body stay healthy when exposed to toxins or stress (Lindberg & Murrell, 2018). Because autophagy is scientifically defined as a renewal process that can take place on a basic cellular level, it has an effect on many processes and manifestations in the physical body that are currently perceived as health issues. These issues include conditions like diabetes, weight problems, cancer, age-related diseases like Alzheimer's and Parkinson disease, and more aesthetic issues like visible signs of aging.

Autophagy has been researched for more than 50 years, and its effects on and benefits of it regarding various types of diseases and health issues have been thoroughly studied. When it was first discovered that a cell would digest or "eat" other cells in the initial research process, researchers didn't understand the reason behind this process and found it to be rather disturbing. However, the research process didn't stop there, and the reason behind this seemingly macabre process and its fantastic restorative and healing results were soon discovered. As you will discover in the book, there are several prominent researchers who dedicated the scientific study of autophagy to different medical and health fields, which include gastroenterology, genome studies, neuropathology, and molecular biology. These are all specialized fields, but the research comes down to studies conducted to inspect the effect of autophagy on the brain, the intestines, and cell production. The best part of all this research is how the studies came to show that autophagy can make us fitter, younger-looking, and more beautiful people, naturally. So, autophagy isn't only about being healthy, but also about discovering the Fountain of Youth and learning how to maintain a healthy weight.

One of the most popular methods used to activate and utilize the benefits of autophagy is through fasting. Fasting has been practiced for thousands of years and for many reasons, including religious ones, and for general wellbeing. It is well-regarded as an ancient practice. Intermittent fasting is a form of intentional fasting as opposed to voluntary fasting, which is associated with starvation (de Cabo & Mattson, 2019). In more modern times, individuals have been experimenting with intermittent fasting and prolonged fasting to reach the level of autophagy. The basic difference between intermittent fasting and prolonged fasting is that intermittent fasting usually consists of shorter fasting periods that cycle with feeding periods, while a prolonged fast can last from 36 hours to a couple of weeks. Intermittent fasting became a "thing" again in the UK after it was introduced in 2012 by the BBC's Horizon documentary *Eat, Fast and Live Longer* (Moseley, 2020). Subsequently, several best-sellers were published, making intermittent fasting a household name. In the United States, intermittent fasting gained popularity in Silicon Valley, and it was the most popular "diet" of 2018 (Solon, 2017). My idea of intermittent fasting involves allowing the body to do its own upkeep. For example, let's say you have a car that you drive a lot. You fill it with gas every other week, but you also occasionally need to take it in for major and minor services and replace certain parts. Imagine if your car were able to service itself, and you only had to do minimal maintenance. This is probably hard to imagine because a car is not biological in any way, but imagine a car had a built-in intelligence that self-regulated and fixed its own issues. All you would have to do is allow this process to occur, and the car would stay young and trendy-looking on the outside. You'd never have to buy a car again! This is the idea I have in my mind about autophagy, and many people are using intermittent fasting to activate autophagy in their bodies in this way to address numerous health reasons.

This book will provide you with all the details about the benefits of autophagy, but it will also provide you with in-depth detail about its research history and how the process of autophagy takes place on a physiological level. By understanding how this cellular process works and how it affects the human body physically, you will be able to utilize it more mindfully by understanding what your body goes through when it is in a state of autophagy, and why you could experience certain symptoms when you decide to use a specific method to reach autophagy, like fasting. Many individuals use fasting to reach a state of autophagy, but they become discouraged easily because of the initial intense hunger sensations they experience. Some think this cannot be healthy, while others find it difficult to persevere, perhaps because of a lack of understanding of the process and what needs to occur before they can reap the ultimate health benefits. Nevertheless, there are countless individuals who swear by autophagy and its benefits and who practice autophagy-activating pursuits daily. So, we'll start with the nitty-gritty history and details about the research that has been conducted, move on to the physiological overview of autophagy, and then we'll start discussing all the perks and hacks plus all the methods you can use to activate autophagy. There are so many benefits to this amazing discovery, and we are now at a place in time where thorough and ongoing research has been conducted on the topic, so there's a lot of information, tips, and tricks that have now been tried and tested as part of this health practice. It's all about learning how to activate the mechanisms in your body and finding the best way for it to fit your practice into your lifestyle.

We don't doubt for a second that our brains are an integral and main form of intelligence in our bodies, and we accept this without question. But, concepts like autophagy that have been researched in-depth and which provide so much enlightening information about the human body proves that it is not only that our minds are intelligent, but that our bodies' intelligence reaches unfathomable depths that extend to a cellular level we never knew existed. Our bodies have evolved to heal and preserve themselves in times of hardship, like those experienced when our ancient ancestors suffered with food shortages or conditions that affected them biologically. This must truly be the most profound superpower discovered in the mechanisms and processing of the human body, and imagine what you'll be missing if you don't learn about and activate your body's own healing, weight-loss, and anti-aging systems!

Chapter 1
Autophagy History and Research

The scientific research field and methodology of autophagy have a long history as studies did not originally include any animal or human being. Even today, most studies in the healthcare industry are being conducted on either yeast or mice as the benefits of autophagy have been identified in these studies, but further conclusive evidence is needed before application can move on to human trials. Understandably. It doesn't matter that all autophagy research has not been conducted on humans, as its amazing effects have been witnessed in fields like nutrition and weight-loss. Scientists had to make several mental leaps to link aspects of autophagy in yeast to an animal or human being because of the fact that autophagy was initially discovered in the cells of yeast. The autophagy research process took more than 50 years, but the results and ongoing research are still astounding. It's hard to imagine, if you consider the hypotheses of some researchers, that the autophagy mechanism has been a part of the human physiological system since we were hunter-gatherers. So much time has gone by since then and we've started changing our eating habits and lifestyles, but our bodies have not shrugged off this process, which means that it must be an integral survival mechanism that we unknowingly deactivated.

In this chapter, we are going to look at the period during which autophagy was first discovered from a scientific perspective and the research process that was subsequently developed. There are many key researchers who have played and still play a role in autophagy research who deserve honorable mention and who can also provide us with an indication of which fields within physiology, disease, health, and medicine the focus has been placed.

The History

Autophagy was discovered more than half-a-century ago, and during that time, researchers used electron microscopes and other biochemical methods. Keith R. Porter and Thomas Ashford observed signs of what would be called autophagy at the Rockefeller Institute in 1962 after examining the liver cells of rats (Ashford & Porter, 1962).

Forty years later, in the 1990s, researchers introduced the field of genetics to autophagy research, and the research potential and development expanded significantly. Using yeast, several groups of scientists, who were working independently, discovered that the yeast contained genes related to autophagy (Takeshige et al., 1992). The genes found in the yeast were given different names, which included APG, AUT, PAG, PAZ, PDD, and GSA. However, in 2003, ATP was chosen by researchers to connote autophagy genes (Klionsky et al., 2003). Beth Levine made a milestone discovery in 1999 by linking autophagy to cancer, and research about this relationship has been flourishing ever since. Autophagy has also been categorized into macroautophagy, microautophagy, and chaperone-mediated autophagy, which we'll be looking at later on.

In 2016, Yoshinori Oshumi received the Nobel Prize for Medicine and Physiology for his in-depth research on several mechanisms related to autophagy. The Nobel Prize was awarded by the Nobel Assembly and the Karolinka Institutet (Fung, 2016a).

Who Coined the Term Autophagy?

The term autophagy was first coined over 50 years ago by C. de Duve. In fact, it was exactly fifty years ago, in 2013. At that stage, the definition of autophagy was the deterioration process of cytoplasmic components in a lysosome, a lysosome being an organelle in a membrane-bound cell that contains digestive enzymes. Although De Duve has since passed away, his terminology has been making waves in the medical and health industry ever since and is now a buzzword in the weight loss industry. The name of the process known as autophagy is derived from a cellular structure called the autophagosome. During the process, the autophagosome becomes a single-membrane structure which is called an autophagolysosome. At this point researchers can observe different stages of organelle degradation. It was through the observation of the process of organelle degradation that De Duve named it autophagy; a name derived from autophagosome and the subsequent autophagolysosome. Thus, autophagy is seen by many as a state that the body enters, but it is actually a process that occurs on a cellular level, and its name refers to this active process (Ohsumi, 2014).

The Focus of Autophagy Research

As mentioned earlier, autophagy research led to a significant development in the research of cancer, but autophagy also made waves in several other fields of medicine and health-related fields. From figuring out the workings of the cellular process to discovering how widespread the function of autophagy actually is, researchers have been studying the effects of autophagy on different diseases, stress and stress-related conditions, the effects of autophagy on blood sugar levels, the effects of autophagy on aging, weight loss, and exercise. Research is ongoing, and papers regarding new developments are regularly published by medical academics. The most important focal point for medical researchers today is research on diseases that exist due to the degeneration of the human brain like Parkinson disease and Alzheimer's and also in-depth studies on how autophagy can be used as a therapeutic and even preventive treatment for different forms of cancer. When I first heard about autophagy, I was really curious and I watched a ton of videos about people who have tried different methods to activate autophagy. However, it's easier to find videos about how autophagy is applied to and what its success rate is on weight loss and fitness than how it was applied to and what its effects were on an illness. I also discovered that research conducted in various healthcare-related fields regarding autophagy is often still in an embryonic stage where hypotheses have been made, and researchers are pretty confident about the outcome of the research, but studies have only been practically conducted on lab rats or mice. This, of course, doesn't refute all the proven benefits of autophagy that promote wellbeing and reduced inflammation in the human body. A lot of studies that include autophagy in their hypotheses utilize intermittent fasting, a combination of intermittent fasting and specific dietary restrictions, and intermittent fasting and physical exercise. When looking at research, fasting appears to be the most popular method of activating autophagy.

Current Researchers and Achievements

Our first researcher to receive honorable mention is Professor Noboru Mizushima. He is a professor at the Department of Biochemistry and Molecular Biology at the University of Tokyo. His major areas of research include the elucidation or clarification of autophagy's mechanisms, the development of methods to monitor autophagy, and the link between autophagy and disease. Mizushima focused on the elucidation of autophagy's mechanisms as part of his research, which included inducing autophagy at the neonatal stage by means of starvation. The implementation of this method showed how important and significant a continued or prolonged state of low-level autophagy is. He also focused his studies on an important component of autophagy research, which is the development of methods for monitoring autophagy. This research was mainly conducted on laboratory mice and rats, where the focus laid on the detection of autophagy, and the development of established methodologies for the assessment and diagnostics of autophagy. Finally, Mizushima focused on the link between autophagy and disease, where he centered his attention on a specific neurodegenerative disease called SENDA (Winning the Nobel Prize Accelerates Clinical Applications of Autophagy, 2020)).

Our next standout is Professor Shigeomi Shimizu, who is a faculty member of the Tokyo Medical and Dental University. He works in the fields of pathological cell biology and pathophysiology. These fields focus on disease, its function, and how its function affects the human body (Pathology, n.d.). Shimizu's discoveries are related to a newly discovered mechanism of autophagy that is called "alternative macroautophagy." This new mechanism is not dependent on DNA that was previously exclusively linked to the autophagy process. His further success is also related to alternative macroautophagy, as his research showed that this mechanism could protect DNA in cells from radiation and the exposure from chemicals. This means that Simizu found a new way autophagy can be utilized in the body and new ways it can be used to protect cells (Winning the Nobel Prize Accelerates Clinical Applications of Autophagy, 2020).

Professor Mamoru Watanabe's focus was not only on pathology and molecular biology, as he also looked at intestinal components related to gastroenterology. He is an Executive Vice-President and researcher at the Tokyo Medical and Dental University. As with much of the research we'll be discussing in this book, Watanabe's is still in the developmental process. Autophagy seems to be a larger and more encompassing physiological concept than any researcher envisioned. Therefore, there are great and promising outcomes to talk about, especially in the medical field, but it is a big fish to fry when talking about sure-fire, tried-and-tested results. So far, Watanabe has discovered that there is a common link between irritable bowel syndrome pathology and autophagy, which opens many doors for further investigation and possible treatment. Studies investigating possible treatment are in the developmental stage as scientists are studying epithelial cells taken from patients during biopsies. If this research yields successful results, this could represent a breakthrough in the treatment of colitis and Chron disease, which causes severe discomfort, pain, and dietary restrictions for patients (Winning the Nobel Prize Accelerates Clinical Applications of Autophagy, 2020).

Professor Hitoshi Okazawa performed some very interesting work regarding autophagy and the brain, and he works at the Medical Research Institute, and also at the Tokyo Medical and Dental University. His fields of expertise are neuropathology and pathophysiology, also known as disordered processes that are linked with injury or disease. Professor Okazawa discovered a way to observe the neural functioning of mice that demonstrated that autophagy could be activated through starvation. The study is also further applied to autophagy's effect on Alzheimer disease. Johji Inazawa is another professor working at the same institute and university who also conducted pioneering research on autophagy, but his focus was cancer. One of the most interesting studies he conducted concerned the relationship between autophagy and cancer stem cells with the aim of finding new therapeutic pathways. He also managed to constitute novel cancer diagnostics and treatments (Winning the Nobel Prize Accelerates Clinical Applications of Autophagy, 2020).

Finally, the researcher who was rewarded for his breakthrough in autophagy research, and also mentioned earlier in the chapter, is Yoshinori Osumi. His breakthrough was specifically based on researching mechanisms for autophagy. Osumi modestly stated that, although his research is conducted on the simplest ingredient; namely, baker's yeast, his hopes were always for his work to have a positive impact on human health.

Now, this is what I'd call interdisciplinary research! All of these individuals, who are experts in their respective medical fields, added the study of autophagy and applied it to our existing and ever-expanding knowledge of the human brain and body. This is possible because the mechanism of autophagy is a fundamental and basic part of human physiology, so it can be applied to many different fields. These are not the only researchers that have made breakthroughs in autophagy, but they have opened new doors by applying the concept and process of autophagy after its basic processes have been studied, documented, and understood by academics.

Chapter 2
Autophagy on a Physiological Level

Now, before we move to all the tips, hacks, and interesting information on how you can become the best version of yourself, let's get sciency for a moment. I'm not the sciency type, at least not on a level where it sounds like a foreign language, but the process of autophagy is actually so interesting that I thought we should give it a try. What I find most interesting is why humans started to, systematically and periodically, move away from the lifestyles that benefited their health the most. I mean, I realize that we tried to make our lives easier and more convenient, and that's something that we do best, but somehow, we neglected or overlooked the essential ways that our bodies work until now. See how I avoided any sciency words there? I went completely philosophical on you! However, now that we know more, why not learn about it? You're going to love it, I promise.

The Process That Leads to Autophagy

It is speculated that autophagy has been present in living organisms for billions of years. The reason why researchers believe this is true is because this mechanism is present in the genomes of every eukaryotic organism in existence. Eukaryotes are organisms that have cells containing a nucleus that is confined with a nuclear envelope. A nucleus is like the brain of a cell because it contains all the genetic goodies. Some organisms that are made of eukaryotes are plants, animals, and fungi, for example. Sounds like almost every living thing, to me. Eukaryotic organisms stand in contrast to prokaryotic organisms that don't have the same cellular structure and are also not associated with autophagy. Examples of prokaryotes can be found in different forms of bacteria. Eukaryotic cells have been the sites of evidence of autophagy and this has been observed by a multitude of researchers. And, that's why scientists first detected the phenomenon and were able to start their research on yeast, as opposed to mammals like lab rats, for example. The fact that they could use yeast as the subject of their study shows us just how integral autophagy is, in not only human existence, but in the existence of most organisms.

As mentioned in the beginning, autophagy can basically be defined as the body's mechanism that gets rid of and recycles all the old "junk" in our body like organelles, cell membranes, and certain proteins; all the components that form part of a cell's mechanics, but which are no longer usable. While we're discussing the process and manifestation of autophagy, it's also important to know that the body has another process it uses that is similar to autophagy called "apoptosis." Apoptosis can also be defined as programmed cell death, and this occurs when cells have divided up until a certain point. This "point" that normally triggers apoptosis will occur when the division of cells is no longer considered healthy, possibly due to cell degradation. Then, apoptosis kicks in to prevent the process of dysfunctional cellular division. The main difference between apoptosis and autophagy is that apoptosis is like a scheduled cell death based on the health of the cell, while the process of autophagy focuses on repairing and reusing different parts within the cell so that it doesn't necessarily have to die or be terminated. Autophagy can also reuse the dead cells to form a collaboration with apoptosis. However, apoptosis, with the aptly-placed "pop" in its name, makes me think of a timer going off, causing blocks of cells to pop like balloons in my body. It is almost as if the cells contain explosive popping candy that's linked to a timer. Imagine walking down the street and experiencing minor pops in your body! At least you would know it's for the sake of your health. Don't know why, but autophagy just seems to be a smoother and more discreet intra-cellular process than this bizarre, surrealistic perspective. Later, the smoothness is going to be discussed on a basic biological level, so you will be able to say "aha!" when we discuss other components like diseases later.

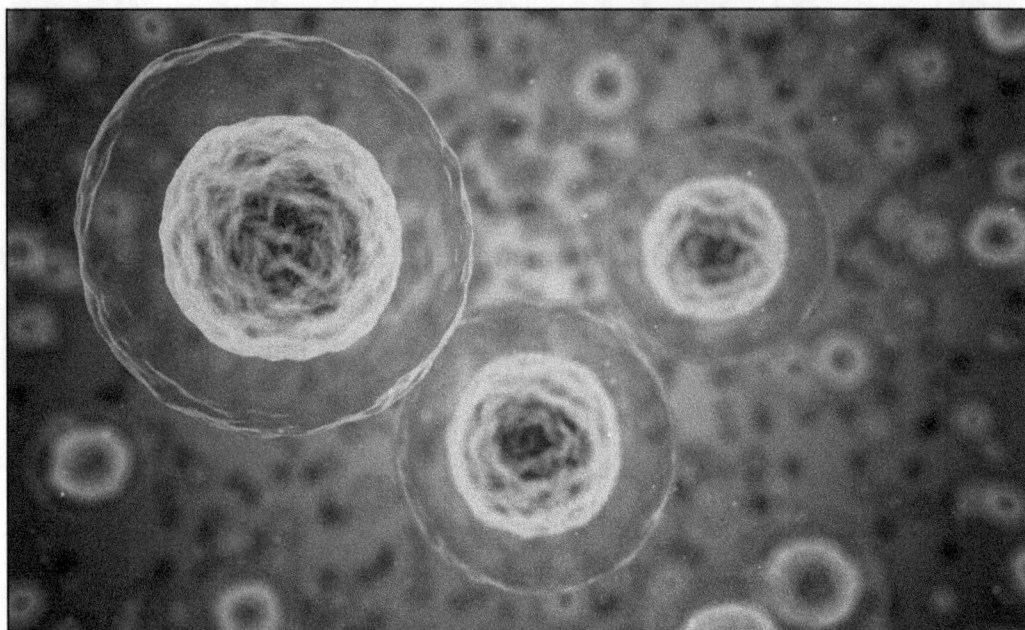

Autophagy On a Cellular Level

The most interesting aspect of autophagy on a cellular level is that it can be both nonselective and selective in its processes. It will, for example, be nonselective when it comes to a case of nutrient deprivation, but selective when it needs to deal with the degradation of organelles and other intracellular components. To recap, the mechanisms of autophagy have been detected in the genomes of eukaryotes, which include mammals, humans, and plants, but not in prokaryotes like bacteria. So, how is this self-digesting mechanism responsible for keeping our bodies clean and functional? Autophagy occurs by the process of biosynthesized lysosomes, and the mechanism of autophagy is related to forming a vesicle or cell with a double membrane that envelopes or encapsulates debris like malformed protein, long-lived or old proteins, cytoplasm, and organelles. This vesicle is known as the autophagosome. After the intra-cellular treasure-hunting is complete, biosynthesis can take place by allowing the vesicle that contains all the dysfunctional material to fuse with a lysosome. Studies indicate that this process has several purposes which include cellular functions like differentiation, growth, organelle turnover, macromolecule turnover, and growth. The process that we discussed above is not as simple as mere treasure-hunting and subsequent synthesis (although that in itself may also not be that simple). For example, when the double-membrane vesicle or cell is formed, 16 different proteins called ATG proteins are required to make this happen. Another need-to-know detail about this process is that it also involves two conjugation systems that are linked with autophagy regulators that will play a determining role in the size and structure or formation of the autophagosome. These proteins and regulators all contribute to the autophagosome's successful fusion with the lysosome, bringing you the ultimate spring-cleaning experience (Levine & Klionsky, 2017; Badadani, 2012). Next, we're going to run through the different types of manifestations of autophagy that each have specific functions in the body for optimal cleansing.

Macroautophagy

Macroautophagy takes a very direct approach to the sequestration of organelles and other cellular components. It is the mainstream mechanism of autophagy that we described above; the removal of parts of cytoplasmic material that can include proteins and organelles within a double-membrane vesicle or body that will, by linking to a lysosome, allow for these materials to degrade. The morphology of macroautophagy is driven by the fact that large parts of the cytoplasm need to be sequestrated instead of more specific parts of a cell, and this is what makes it such a unique process (Klionsky & Codogno, 2013).

Microautophagy

Microautophagy seems to be the most complicated process of the three and focuses on the transport of cytosolic components by enwrapping them in what is called lysosomal membrane dynamics. Microautophagy has, after extensive studies, been classified into 3 types. The first type is microautophagy with lysosomal protrusion. Next up is microautophagy with endosomal invagination, and finally, microautophagy with endosomal invagination. All 3 types have been studied in mammalian cells, plant cells, and in yeast cells. These microautophagic pathways can be understood by firstly categorizing them in terms of morphology, which includes protrusion or invagination, and, secondly location, which translates to the vacuole of the endosome or the lysosome regarding their membrane dynamics. Finally, another interesting factoid about microautophagy is that it can be selective or nonselective (Oku & Sakai, 2018). But, let's stop there as we are about to move one to our final point, chaperone-mediated autophagy, before we'll start to discuss the ways you can invoke these beneficial cellular processes.

Chaperone-Mediated Autophagy

This method of autophagy is called "chaperone-mediated" because it refers to the specific chaperone-dependent cytosolic proteins, which are what chaperone-mediated autophagy targets for transport and degradation. Chaperone-mediated autophagy transports the cytosolic proteins to targeted lysosomes and has the ability to directly translocate the protein across the lysosome's membrane for the degradation process (Kaushik & Cuervo, 2012). This is terrible, as it makes me think of taking someone's hand and leading them directly into a trap. I guess these old cytosolic proteins have seen better days if they are being chaperoned across the lysosome border. At least the process will make me look younger and feel healthier as a result.

Chapter 3
Fasting for Weight Loss

What do you do when you feel hungry? Probably what most of us do; you rationalize and motivate the need for eating something, and then you eat it. But, what if I were to tell you that you should react by inwardly shouting, "Shut up, you darned hormones!" instead of rationalizing every single hunger pang? Is your body always in need of nourishment when you feel like eating something? If not, then why do you feel hungry? The human body is so smart that it may seem to be too smart sometimes. That hunger pang you feel most of the time is not your body ready to collapse due to a lack of nourishment. It's your brain, secreting the hunger hormone *ghrelin* on the basis of habit, reminding you to eat. Have you noticed that you tend to be hungry at the same time every day, even if your eating pattern is not completely consistent? That's your brain behaving in its most primal state, terrified that you're going to starve to death when the opposite is actually true.

The most well-known method of activating autophagy is through the practice of fasting. The practice of fasting also includes intermittent fasting, where fasting is practiced at specific times and alternated with periods of eating. Intermittent fasting can be simply defined by a schedule that consists of eating and fasting periods. This means that for a specific time of the day, an individual would have an "eating window" where they could nourish their bodies with food, and the rest of the day would be spent fasting, which means that no food would be consumed. The focus of intermittent fasting for weight loss that makes it so popular is that it's not a diet per se; there are no strict rules telling you what to eat, so all your focus is on sticking to the eating and fasting schedules (Intermittent Fasting 101 — The Ultimate Beginner's Guide, 2020). These fasting and eating timeframes are known as fasting and feeding windows that help regulate different processes in your body and aid digestion.

The fasting process is seen to be a natural part of human evolution and an integral component of how our bodies developed from our hunter-gatherer ancestors. If you think about it, our ancient ancestors did not have access to supermarkets and handy gadgets like refrigerators, so their bodies needed to adapt to keep themselves going and healthy until they found their next meal. This is why our bodies, although we may not believe it, can function without food for much longer than we think. And, looking at the history of our ancestors and their eating habits, incorporating the occasional fasting period into your week provides your body with a more natural way to function than when eating 3 or more meals a day (Intermittent Fasting 101 — The Ultimate Beginner's Guide, 2020). Fasting is also practiced in several different religions, including Buddhism, Islam, and Christianity, but in this chapter, we'll be focusing on a non-religious approach that investigates the health benefits we have to gain from intermittent fasting.

Intermittent Fasting

Has someone you know ever expressed their opinion about fasting by comparing it to starvation? Alternatively, have you ever started talking about intermittent fasting only to be interrupted by someone who tries to convince you that it's unhealthy and that "the body needs food regularly to be able to function?" I wish that I had a nickel for every time I've heard that! These are common misconceptions, mostly uttered by individuals who've heard about intermittent fasting, but who haven't done any research or reading on the topic. Maybe they dismissed the idea immediately because it sounded like too much of an inconvenience. Before you sit back and agree with them, take a look at the benefits of intermittent fasting, as they are plentiful.

There are several popular intermittent fasting methods or timeframes, but you don't have to stick to one religiously to get the results you want. However, using them as guidelines is a great way to know when you should be feeding and when you should be fasting, and that is why they are so popular. Before we start looking at the different fasting schedules, their benefits, and how they can be applied, it's important to understand what happens inside the body during the fasting window and how fasting activates processes like fat-burning and autophagy. Reaching autophagy through fasting takes a while, but the body reaches different stages that are important to know about from the beginning of a fasting window until the time you decide to end it. These stages also have major health benefits, so it's not like you're wasting your time waiting for the "hour of autophagy" to begin.

The concept behind activating autophagy with fasting is to put the body in a stressed state that is considered "healthy" (Yu, 2020). Is there such a thing? Well, in life, we are able to discern between healthy stress and unhealthy or toxic stress, so for the body to be hungry while it still has a myriad of reserves it can use is probably not a form of unhealthy stress. Compare a body in a fasted state to a body that has a common cold. Which effect do you think causes toxic stress on the body? While the common cold causes inflammation, a fasted state will eventually lead to decreased inflammation, which makes fasting a healthy stressor and being sick a toxic type of stress. Putting the body under healthy stress by fasting activates autophagy, which is the natural way the body adapts and responds to stress (Yu, 2020).

The first zero to six hours of a fasting period is seen as a fed state because your body is still busy dealing with your last meal. You know; absorbing nutrients, large-scale digestive activities, and so on. After having your last meal before entering a fasting window, your glucose levels will rise because of the caloric intake and will stimulate the production and secretion of insulin. When the body produces insulin, it signals for protein integration, which means that glucose moves into the cells as a source of energy. Also, any excess glucose moves to the liver for storage and remains there until the body needs it for energy. However, the liver has a glucose storage limit, and as soon as this limit is reached, the leftover glucose is stored as fat. This process, where glucose is converted into fat, is called *lipogenesis* (Coulson, 2020). What this means is that, during the first 6 hours of your fast, your body is still dealing with the unfinished business of your last meal and wrapping things up so that it can move on to the next stage. That is, if you don't decide to eat something or consume anything that will trigger insulin production. So far, so good.

After six hours, things start to happen. The glucose level in the blood starts to decrease, and this subsequently leads to a decrease in the production of insulin. Your body's natural response is to move back to those glycogen stores in your liver and to use them as a source of energy, so the liver starts to break down the glucagon to produce energy. Now, if you've reached the 12-hour mark, then it means that your body has finished most of the digesting and processing of your last meal and can now enter a resting phase. Now, your body can finally start to focus on healing while increasing the level of human growth hormone in its system. At this stage, glucagon is also released from your liver to help stabilize your blood sugar. This is where the fat-burning process kicks into gear. For the next six hours, you can sit back, relax, and experience a consistent rise in your human growth hormone levels accompanied by consistent fat burning (Coulson, 2020).

If you decide that you want to make it to or past the 18-hour mark, you have some more treats coming your way. At 18 to 20 hours, your body's autophagy will activate, and ketones will be released. From there on, most individuals who practice intermittent fasting will decide to close their fasting window, but if you extend it up to 36 hours, the levels of autophagy in your body will increase to 300%. As a bonus, if you extend your fast to 48 hours, your body will spontaneously start its own cell-renewal process as well as reduce inflammation. Finally, if you want your autophagy to peak, you can extend a healthy fast to 72 hours (Coulson, 2020).

As you can see here, intermittent fasting for weight loss is built more around the fat-burning benefits than the full-blown regenerative miracles of autophagy because of how long a fasting window is required to be for the body to clean all those hard-to-reach places. The fat-burning benefits come first and are then followed by the growth hormone and cell regeneration, which can take three to four days. That's why we're looking at the weight-loss component and the other health benefits separately because they require different fasting or autophagy-activation methods to be their most successful. For fasting that prioritizes weight loss, there are several popular fasting regimes we'll be looking at. They are the 14/10, 16/8, 20/4, 5:2, and alternate day fasting. Not everyone is built the same, so some may have different fasting times and durations that work for them. To find out what may work for you, let's look at all of them in more detail:

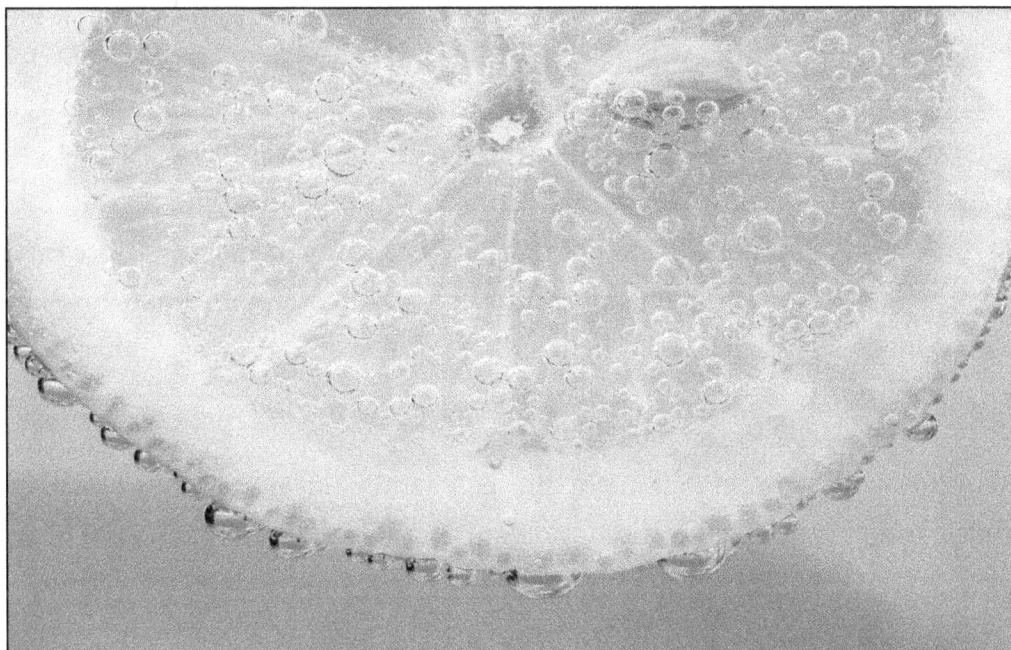

The Circadian Rhythm

A person's circadian rhythm is considered to be a natural internal clock that regulates their metabolism, but there is also something called the "Circadian Rhythm Diet." Your circadian rhythm is probably the most natural way for your body to know what it needs by being sensitive to light, melanin, and other factors. It is your internal clock, and it is also known as your sleep/

wake cycle. When we don't maintain a consistent sleeping pattern or don't sleep enough, this can affect two specific hormones that are linked to our appetite. They are ghrelin, which makes you feel hungry and leptin, which makes you feel full. When you are overtired, your body will increase ghrelin levels, which will make you feel increasingly hungry when you actually don't need any food (Nazish, 2020).

The circadian rhythm is the maternal foundation of modern-day intermittent fasting because it is mainly based on when you eat as opposed to how much or what you eat. Also known as the "body clock diet," your eating times are restricted, just like with more intense versions of intermittent fasting. In fasting terms, it's basically a 12/12, and it's supposed to coordinate with the daytime/nighttime ratio. Your feeding window is during the daytime, and your fasting window is after dark until dawn. Dieticians recommend that you focus on breakfast and lunch being your bigger meals and eating a light dinner before it gets dark. Because the feeding window is larger than other types of intermittent fasting, there is more time to divide up your calories, so you don't need to eat large meals. The rationale behind this eating pattern is that our metabolisms are closely linked to our circadian rhythm; hence, the fact that it can influence the secretion of our hunger hormones (Nazish, 2020).

Working with your circadian rhythm is a gentle and natural approach, so this is the first step in our discussion about intermittent fasting. It is, however, not as well-known among the fasting community as other methods. Next, we're going to look at the basic 14/10, which is a common starting point for new fasters.

14/10

The 14/10 method is a lot like the 12/12 or the circadian rhythm. It is a relatively easy fasting schedule and with the 14/10, it just means that you will be in a fasting state for 14 hours and then enter a feeding state of 10 hours. This method is a great way to get started because you can design your fasting and feeding windows in such a way that most of the fasting will happen while you are sleeping. If you decide to follow or start with the 14/10 method, you can help yourself adjust gradually towards longer fasting periods by fasting during the time of day when you are the least hungry. For example, if you aren't really hungry in the morning, you can start your fast at 8:00 or 9:00 in the evening, which means you will enter your feeding window the next morning at 10:00 or 11:00. So, instead of eating some cereal when you wake up, you can have some black coffee or tea, which doesn't affect your insulin levels, and plan a nice meal for when your fasting window ends. This fasting option will give you a taste of what intermittent fasting is like while introducing your body to activating its own fat-burning mechanisms. You can, however, upgrade or lengthen your fasting period for better results. The 14/10 schedule is for individuals who are physiologically most likely not able to do intense fasting and for those who want to get their bodies accustomed to the fasting experience.

16/8

The 16/8 method is probably the most commonly used fasting method for weight loss because it still has reasonable feeding and fasting windows while also fitting into most people's lifestyles while showing positive results. In other words or fewer words, it's the "best of everything" option. The most common way the 16/8 is applied is by also placing most of the fasting hours during nighttime so that the only meal that needs skipping would be breakfast. For example, you can apply 16/8 by starting your fast at 8:00 or 9:00 in the evening, which means that your first meal the next day will be at 12:00 or 1:00 in the afternoon, respectively. Sounds reasonable, right? The trick is though, that while you are fasting, you can't consume anything to "lift" your blood sugar levels like coffee with milk and sugar or soda, as this will break the fast, meaning you will have to start all over again. This is mainly where people struggle. You may be someone who doesn't usually eat in the morning, but who grabs a cappuccino, but now, from a fasting perspective, that cappuccino cannot be consumed until noon, or it will have to be swapped for a water or black coffee. Otherwise, it will break the fast you've been working on so hard all night in your sleep. This is an important point to keep in mind while fasting; it's better not to snack and to avoid liquid calories to ensure that your fast is effective. But don't worry, we'll get into detail about this shortly.

20/4 "The Warrior Diet"

This fasting time frame is meant for warriors because your eating window is only four hours long, while your fasting window is twenty hours long. If you want to level-up your warrior status, you can even do a 24/0 where you literally eat one meal a day and fast the rest of the time. If you have an active social life or have a large family, maintaining the 20/4 on a daily basis may be more difficult because you won't be able to take part in all the eating- and drinking-centered activities that are part of modern culture. This fasting regime is for a person who wants to focus on health and weight loss and push the other aspects of life aside for a while. Individuals who follow the 20/4 method usually take their feeding window in the late morning or afternoon. For example, a good time to have your meal would be between 1:00 and 5:00 in the afternoon, or even a bit earlier or later. Prolonging your fasting period gives your body time to do more restorative tasks and burn extra fat (Fung & Scher, 2020).

5:2

The 5:2 is the next method we're going to discuss that works somewhat differently from fasting methods like 16/8 and 20/4, where you enter shorter fasting and feeding windows on a daily basis. In this method, you get to follow a normal eating pattern for five days and then will fast for two days or 48 hours. However, during this long fast, you are allowed to eat 500 calories each day, which you can either eat in one meal or spread out into small low-calorie snacks (Fung & Scher, 2020). Think vegetables, green smoothies, and foods that provide vitamins and nourishment for your body, but in tiny quantities. This method is also one of the fasting methods that carry more scientific support than others, but it is difficult to stick to this method exactly because you'll be fasting for a full 48 hours. For example, would you designate your two fasting days on the weekend or endure them when you're working during the week? It's a tough call, but there's definitely a pot of gold at the end of the rainbow.

Alternate Day Fasting

The alternate day fasting method appears to achieve the best results of weight loss, promising quick results. This method entails eating normally every other day and fasting on the days in between. On your fasting days, you can consume 500 calories to nourish your body, but you can also do a clean fast with no calories at all. Some individuals find alternate day fasting easier than the 5:2 method. This may be because you won't be sinking back into the habit of eating normally for so long before having to enter a prolonged fasting window. Many studies have been conducted on this fasting method that provide us with some helpful tips and guidelines. For example, if you want to follow this method, then the decision between doing a clear fast and a restricted caloric intake on your fasting days will not affect the effectiveness of your weight loss. Additionally, the way you "spread" your 500 calories on your fasting days will also not affect your weight loss potential in this eating plan (Bjarnadottir et al., 2020). This is great news!

When it comes to hunger, you may be one of the lucky ones who automatically develops a new neural pathway that reduces those hunger pangs on a fasting day and brings them back up to normal on a feeding day. However, some individuals following this eating pattern have indicated that their hunger levels don't change at all. Maybe it's a mindset thing? (Bjarnadottir et al., 2020).

OMAD

If you do an OMAD, you're a badass. This fasting schedule should definitely not be one of the beginner options, as what you put in your mouth is actually important because, using this method, you would only eat once a day. OMAD stands for "one meal a day," and this meal is usually consumed at lunch because it is relatively big and should be calorie- and nutrient-dense. So, what you'll be doing is fasting for 23 hours, and giving yourself a one-hour feeding window. This doesn't mean you should stuff different types of junk food down your gullet for the entire hour though. If you become an OMAD fan, your stomach is not going to like it. The reason OMAD followers like this routine is because it is so simple and minimalistic. Eating seems to be a hassle for them, if you ask me, so they do it once a day, requiring less meal-scheduling and less meal-prepping. However, you need to consume ALL of your required calories in that one meal to stay healthy (Jockers, 2019).

So, when should you break your OMAD fast? Medical professionals say that the best time for your body and your social life is between 4:00 and 7:00 p.m. Personally, I'd want to break my fast around lunchtime, so I guess it depends from person to person. If you need some guidelines about how your meal should look and what it should consist of, you can focus on foods that contain healthy fats to make up for your daily calorie needs. Secondly, you will need to focus on nutrient density and add in quality protein, vegetables, and healthy carbs to your meal. Try to use one normal-sized plate, but don't worry about stacking it; you can pile your food up to three inches high. Don't be shy! Finally, sticking to a balanced meal instead of trying to make up the calories with junk food is going to considerably improve the way you feel. If you want to eat for an entire hour, make sure it's all spent on that plate of food. Finally, while you need to hydrate while you are in your fasting window, try to drink as little as possible during your small feeding window. You won't want to fill up your stomach with liquid or dilute the digestive liquids you need to process your meal. Even a glass of red wine is recommended. Enjoy (Jockers, 2019).

Keep This in Mind

You might have heard somewhere that, when practicing intermittent fasting, the focus is not on what you eat and how much you eat like with usual diets or eating plans, as these are not the focal points of the intermittent fasting plan or model. There are, however, good reasons why one shouldn't binge before or after a fast and overindulge on junk food and candy, so intermittent fasting should not be used as an excuse to overindulge every time you enter a feeding window. Let's take a look at some important tips and hacks that will bring you successful intermittent fasting for weight loss.

The first tip that will really help you get through those initial fasting windows where you experience extreme hunger is to stay hydrated and fill your stomach with water. If you feel that you are experiencing a slump due to your body adjusting to the new routine, a great go-to is a black coffee or tea. Coffee specifically gets rave-reviews by hardcore fasters and, if you drink it without the cream and sugar in a fasted state, it even has some health benefits, which include mental clarity and the acceleration of autophagy. Next, we have to deal with what to do when you get those hunger pangs and need-to-eat urges. There's no other way than to tough it out. But, you can make it easier on yourself by not sitting and thinking about it constantly. Try to stay busy and schedule some have-to-get-done work for these times. If you start getting into your work or whatever you decided to do, chances are you'll forget about the hunger. I know it's easier said than done, but it's possible, and it'll happen sooner than you think. Working from home can really make it hard to maintain a regular and healthy eating schedule or pattern because the fridge is just around the corner. When I worked in an office, I never had any change for the vending machine, so I'd just go to the kitchen and make myself a cup of coffee. We have to be strong and be the rulers of our environment! When that hunger pang starts to irritate you, ask yourself, "Is my wellbeing, health, or life on the line if I don't eat something right now?" I know; pretty dramatic, but it's a valid question nonetheless. Wait it out, ride the wave, and you'll see that hunger disappear as quickly as it reared its ugly head. And, you'll feel accomplishment that is well-deserved. After all this talk of mental strength, let's also talk about the fact that you may need assistance in the beginning to take the edge off, so when you decide to start intermittent fasting, you can keep the following items in stock, apart from coffee and water:

Green tea is a great way to accelerate your metabolism and to help you fight off the most agonizing hunger pangs. You also don't have to wait for the hunger to set in before boiling the kettle; you can make a cup of green tea part of your fasting routine. You can also keep chia seeds in your pantry for those days when you feel like your stomach is contracting with emptiness. Soaking the chia seeds in water for thirty minutes creates a fiber-rich gel-like substance that will fill the hole in your stomach until you enter your feeding window and chia seeds provide nutritional benefits like Omega-3 fatty acids. Finally, you can consider adding cinnamon to your tea or coffee as it may provide some extra appetite suppression. Cinnamon also has a positive effect on your blood sugar levels, which can help accelerate the weight-loss process (Fung & Scher, 2020). In a world that bombards us with food, and delicious food for that matter, we sometimes need to take a step back for the sake of our health.

Now, after we've discussed controlling your hunger during fasting windows, let's look at how you can increase the effectiveness of your intermittent fasting venture by carefully choosing what to eat during your feeding windows. I know that a popular selling point for intermittent fasting is the "you can still eat what you want" catchphrase, but the process your body undergoes during fasting can cause you to feel quite uncomfortable if you decide to go on a junk food binge after fasting, especially if you eat a lot of foods with high sugar content. By lowering your carb intake during your feeding windows, you will not only make your fasting journey more effective, but fasting will also become easier and more natural for your body because you won't cause unnecessary insulin spikes during your feeding windows. Remember that, when you fast, your body regulates and lowers your blood sugar levels and insulin production accordingly, so if you decide to eat a whole box of donuts after fasting, the sugar spike will leave you feeling hungover and alienated from the intermittent fasting process. This doesn't mean that you need to restrict yourself completely; the point of fasting is to give you more dietary freedom. But, moderation is key. Have one piece of cake, eat it, enjoy it, and move on to bluer skies (Fung & Scher, 2020).

When you reach the end of your fasting window, assess your hunger level. Are you ravenous, or is your hunger actually psychological? You know, you are so in the habit of eating that it feels strange to not eat for so long, so now you want to make up for that period of abstinence (Fung & Scher, 2020). And allow yourself to be honest. If it's the second option, you've taken a massive step forward towards improving your health by identifying why you have the need to eat most of the time. Fasting and intermittent fasting have the ability to bring you back to a level where your body can intuitively identify real hunger, which means that your need to eat is based on your body's requirement of nutrients and for sustenance. This is the healthiest reason to eat, not to mention the most rational! If this is your main reason for eating and you save treating yourself for special occasions, then the weight will seem to melt off. Allowing your body to reset back to its most natural form can also reduce your need to indulge and overeat if you let your mind allow it. So, let's get back to breaking your fast. The best way to do it is in a gentle and caring way so as not to overload your digestive system and cause discomfort. For example, you can go green with a nutritious smoothie or eat a handful of almonds or a salad (Fung & Scher, 2020). Your stomach will thank you, and you will feel invigorated.

The Dirt on Dirty Fasting

If you don't prefer your fasting routine to be saintly and all-white, you can always turn on your naughty side and give dirty fasting a try. Does it work? That's what we're here to discuss, so let's dig in and get dirty.

When you look at the definition of dirty fasting, it becomes even clearer how saintly clean fasting really is. This is because, to be labeled a dirty faster, the only thing you need to do differently is to drink diet soda or add artificial sweeteners to your coffee as these are considered to be possible insulin or blood sugar triggers which, according to the traditional (clean) fasting dogma, will prevent your body from reaching autophagy in the intended timeframe. A "dirty faster" will tell you that artificial sweetener doesn't necessarily have an impact on your insulin responses and I think that that's the main difference between the saints and the dirties. The saints want to make extra sure and take all the precautions necessary to ensure a successful and clean fast, while the dirties don't care about taking a risk here and there, as long as the main component, mainly food, is avoided during a fasting window. So, what do our dirties see as acceptable beverages during a fasting window? This can range from bulletproof or sweetened coffee to diet soda, to sugar-free gum. But do they lose weight? Only some do (Beaver, 2019). If you ask me, by introducing components that can trigger an insulin response during your fasting window, you will be taking the risk of foregoing the fat-burning and other health benefits of fasting, which would bring you back to a diet dependent on calorie restriction. This may be why this method works for some and not for others; it may depend on what you eat in your feeding window and if you incorporate physical activity along with your dirty fasting approach.

Chapter 4
Getting Physical

How do you feel about fasted exercise? Do you think it can be productive or even possible? I've discussed the idea with one or two people, and they found it unfathomable. "But you have no fuel in your body; how are you going to exercise if you have no energy?" That was their response in a nutshell. This is one of those cases where the capabilities of autophagy are going to blow your socks off again and not for the last time either. It is a well-known fact that exercise can activate autophagy in your body, but what if you combine exercise with fasting? Will it be hard? Can you develop and build muscle effectively, and will it accelerate weight loss? People are doing it and raving about it. But, let's look at the facts. We are all different and our bodies have different requirements, whether they be nutritional or otherwise. Let's start by looking at the conventional advice for active individuals.

Autophagy, Exercise, and Fasting

Many fitness gurus and personal trainers recommend eating a small meal before a workout that your body can use as fuel. However, this may leave you feeling heavy or sluggish and can affect effectiveness during your workout. The recommendation of fasted exercise has been on the rise during the past few years, but there are differing opinions about the intensity one should maintain while exercising in a fasted state. Many health professionals, including doctors, recommend, in written and published articles, exercise during fasting as it has the potential to activate an enhanced state of autophagy, boost anti-aging, and rev up your fat burning to a new level. This means that, if you exercise in a fasted state regularly, you can improve your level of insulin sensitivity, and this can lead to increased production of the human growth hormone that helps you get all those desired effects, including weight loss, effective fat-burning, and muscle building or maintenance (Jockers, 2019).

Increased Fat Burning

Because your body is in a fasted state, it is already reaching for reserves within your body for fuel. By adding fasted exercise, you can accelerate this process to the point where your body depletes its glycogen stores from the liver and starts burning ketones. By making fasted exercise a habit, you can develop what is called energy efficiency, which means that your body will be using its energy in the most efficient way possible for proper bodily function. It also develops another potent function called metabolic flexibility, which means the body has developed the ability to adapt to the environment by changing its metabolism (Jockers, 2019).

Tips for Efficient Fasted Exercise

Applying exercise while fasting is very beneficial, and you're going to see definite results, but like with fasting, you're going to have to ease into it and not put too much stress on your body at first. Like we discussed earlier, fasting is a type of stress, and even though it's a healthy type of stress, one needs to be cautious when increasing the stress level. For example, you may want to consult your physician before making a big change in your lifestyle, and even then, consider easing into a fasting routine first before gradually adding exercise. On the other hand, if you exercise regularly and yet are new to fasting, you may only need to turn it down a few notches in the beginning and slowly work up to your usual level again.

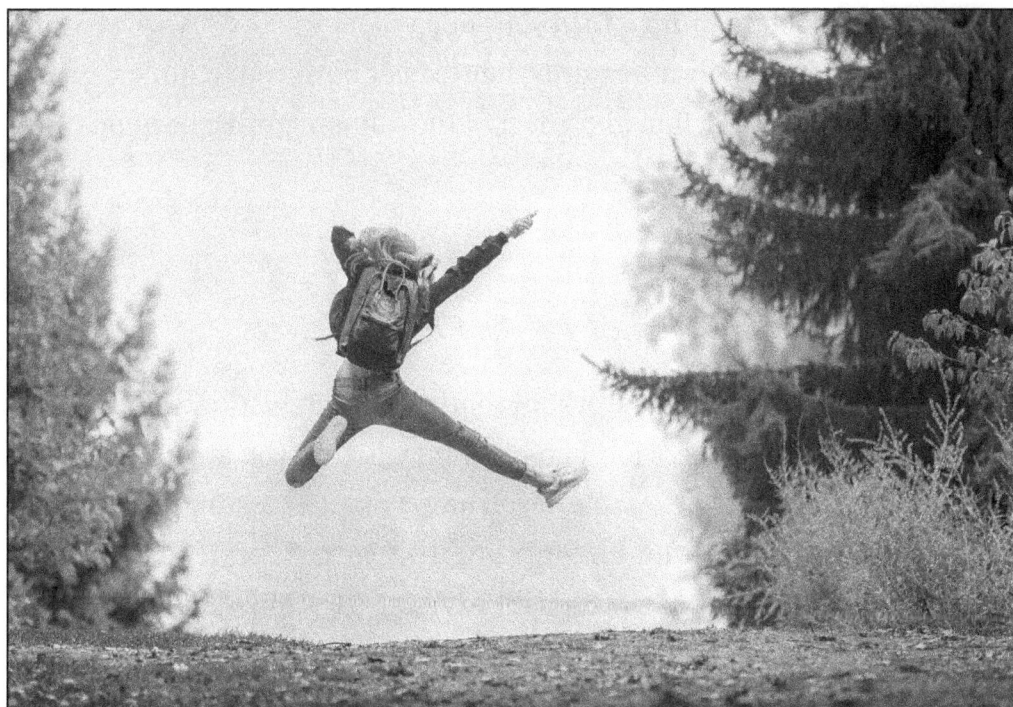

The first thing you can do to maximize your efforts and results is to exercise at the end of your fasting window. If you can't manage to do this, it doesn't mean that you won't get any benefits from fasted exercise. However, keep in mind that, at the end of your fasting window, you will have reached the peak of your fasting period, which means that adding exercise at that point will render the best results. Next, keep in mind that your body is going to need an adequate amount of rest and nutrition to support this active lifestyle. Not that your body doesn't need it anyway, but when exercising in a fasted state, you can love and nourish your body by focusing on nutrient-dense, whole foods (Jockers, 2019). Feast on protein, healthy fats, and unrefined carbs to replenish and restore what's needed during your feeding window. Your main go-to guidelines for fasted exercise are to always stay hydrated, to choose high-intensity training, but not exceed thirty minutes of exercise, and to consume a good quality protein source and a source of BCAA's after training to help with the recovery process. BCAA's, or branched-chain amino acids, consist of mostly essential amino acids your muscles need for recovery and growth. You can also take BCAA's before your workout in the form of a pre-workout drink or supplement if your focus is specifically to build muscle. A final pro-tip is to, if you supplement with BCAA's post-work-out, not eat immediately afterwards, but to wait until you're hungry as this will increase the production and effect of the human growth hormone even more (Jockers, 2019).

Fasted Exercise Strategies for All Fitness Levels

If you decide to start a fasted workout routine, the intensity of your workout will depend on your fitness level and also on whether you are a beginner at intermittent fasting. For example, if you are a complete fasting newbie, your best bet will be to start with a short 12 to 14-hour fast combined with light cardio that you can alternate with light resistance training. By starting light and easy, the routine won't feel unattainable to you, and you can gradually increase your intensity if you choose to do so. If you are at an intermediate level or you feel that you're ready to move up from your beginner's fasting position, you can try a 14 to 16-hour fast combined with high-intensity interval training or HIIT and alternate it with high-intensity resistance training or HIRT. If you choose to follow this routine, you would want to already be getting the hang of intermittent fasting. It's definitely going to get the blood pumping through your veins. Finally, if you are at an advanced fitness level and no stranger to intermittent fasting, there are two ways you can choose to go. The first way is an advanced fat-burning method, and the second is an advanced muscle-building method. They both contain the same exercise components, but are performed in a different sequence. For example, for muscle gain, your ultimate recipe for success is to fast from anything between 16 and 24 and to combine it with a routine that starts with HIRT and ends with HIIT. However, if you want to burn those pesky extra inches or maintain your physique with an advanced fat-burning routine, your go-to would be the same fasting routine, but it would be followed by a HIIT-HIRT sequence. In both of these cases, it is best to keep your exercise regime under five or exactly five sessions a week to make sure that you don't over train or exhaust your body (Jockers, 2019).

Once you get into the fasted training routine, you may enjoy it so much when you start seeing results that you start overtraining. It's important to monitor your stress levels, sleeping patterns, and how your immune system copes with the environment because this can be an indication of overtraining. If you experience excessive soreness in your muscles, irritability, fatigue, anxiety, nutrient deficiencies, or joint pain, you may be suffering from overtraining, and you need to give your body a break (Jockers, 2019). Step it down a notch and perhaps focus the purpose of your training on stress relief and mood improvement instead of reaching a specific fitness goal for that period of time. In other words, focus on working out for fun. Not that it's not fun otherwise, but you know what I mean. Work out to feel refreshed and energized at the end instead of wasted and sore and do this in whichever way works best for you and your body. If you want to pause your fasted workouts and work out during your feeding window while your body and mind recover, then go for it. Intermittent fasters are usually more in tune with their bodies' needs than non-fasters, so you'll know if you need to see a physician, take a few days off, or just take it easy. Eat well, sleep well, and make time to relax and do what you enjoy doing.

The Myth of Fasting, Autophagy, and Muscle Loss

When we spoke about intermittent fasting earlier in the chapter, we differentiated between involuntary fasting and intentional fasting. Intermittent fasting is a type of intentional fasting where an individual sets up specific times for abstinence and feeding. On the other hand, involuntary fasting is linked to starvation, where there is no set time frame for fasting and eating. When it comes to the loss of muscle mass, these two fasting types are like day and night. Because involuntary fasting can last for any amount of time, there is no feeding process that provides restoration, which means conservation of the body doesn't take place. If this does not happen and prolonged fasting turns into starving, the body will start using its own muscle mass for energy. However, in the case of intermittent fasting, the results of studies conducted specifically on intermittent fasting and muscle loss, indicate the opposite effect (Tinsley, 2017).

One study indicated that inhibiting autophagy during a fasting or even a starving process intensified muscle loss. Because autophagy flow is crucial to maintain the integrity of myofibers, it is just as important to preserve muscle mass (Masiero et al., 2009). In a 2010 study that included alternate day fasting, patients were set on a normal eating schedule alternating with a fasting day. The results of this study were that patients were able to lose body fat, but that they did not suffer any loss of muscle mass. This study was followed up with a more recent one in 2016, where a different strategy was followed to test muscle loss in patients. In this study, participants were divided into two groups. One group was placed on an intermittent fasting schedule while the other group followed a normal calorie-restricted diet. The outcome was quite surprising. The percentage of the lean mass of the fasting group increased by 2.2%, while the percentage of the lean mass in the calorie-restricted diet group increased by 0.5%. This suggests that intermittent fasting can be up to four times more effective at preserving lean muscle mass. These studies also showed other important factors that separate calorie-restricted diets from intermittent fasting. For example, intermittent fasting enables your body to "switch fuel sources," while a significant calorie restriction can cause your body to shut down. Switching fuel sources means that your body is going to switch to burning fat and doing some spring cleaning, which means that fasting keeps your body in a highly functional state. Another very interesting conclusion garnered from this study is that calorie restriction will ultimately increase the secretion of ghrelin, which is the "hungry" hormone. Intermittent fasting ultimately suppresses this hormone, making you feel less hungry, probably because your body is still feeding - just not on food (Fung, 2018).

If you had any doubts about losing muscle while fasting, then rest assured, as science rules in your favor.

Chapter 5
Autophagy's Amazing Effects on Disease

Autophagy research did not only cover weight loss, but researchers found that this mechanism in the human body is so intelligent and is such an inherent part of our physiological functioning that it affects almost every aspect of the human body in terms of health. Researchers started conducting studies regarding specific health conditions and diseases that, in each of their degradative physiological processes, can hypothetically link to the healing process of autophagy. For example, scientists discovered the astounding effect that autophagy has on brain health. This means that studying a disease like Alzheimer's, which is characterized by cognitive and neural decline, can bring new answers if linked to autophagy studies. Some complicated research cases were identified at the beginning of this book along with the professors who conducted them. The fact that those researchers are already investigating and researching such a wide variety of ailments and the effect of autophagy on many parts of our physiology indicates a promising future for healthcare. We have, for such an incredibly long time, been told to take medication for different ailments and this has become the norm, based on research and successful trials. I'm not saying that we all need to throw our meds out of the window. There is a reason why a medical specialist prescribed them for you. However, self-healing or placing the body in a state where you enable it to create or support homeostasis without external help is ideal. It seems that, in our pursuit of health and longevity, we have moved our focus in some way to a more natural approach, maybe to discover mechanisms that can work in tandem with pharmaceutical medication. Before we go any further, it's also important to note that the incredible amount of knowledge that has been discovered recently shows that we still know very little about the human body, and when reading about all of the research discussed here, I think it may be a smart choice to keep in mind that this may not be the end of the story and that new research may still be uncovered. For all we know, this is the beginning. However, that does not in any shape or form suggest that we cannot start educating ourselves right now.

Autophagy's Healing Perks

When it comes to disease and medical issues, a weight-loss approach like intermittent fasting may not always be successful. One needs to consider the nature of each ailment, its symptoms, cause, and what needs to happen during the autophagy process in order to achieve improved health and effective results. These methods are definitely not as clear and well-researched as the ones that are tried and tested for weight loss and exercise alone, but research is in process and we can share what we currently know, which is definitely not discouraging. When we discussed the process of fasting and how the process is used to induce autophagy, it was clear that it can take quite a while—for some even longer than others. So, if you suffer from a specific condition, how long does your body need to be in an autophagic state to receive a satisfactory, therapeutic effect? Maybe there are other ways to induce autophagy for certain cases of illness. In the discussion which follows, there are unanswered questions, but there is also hope.

Cholesterol

Most of us know someone who suffers from high cholesterol; it's like it's not even a big deal anymore. People's main objective is just to get through their day and get things done while not really focusing on their health. Could this

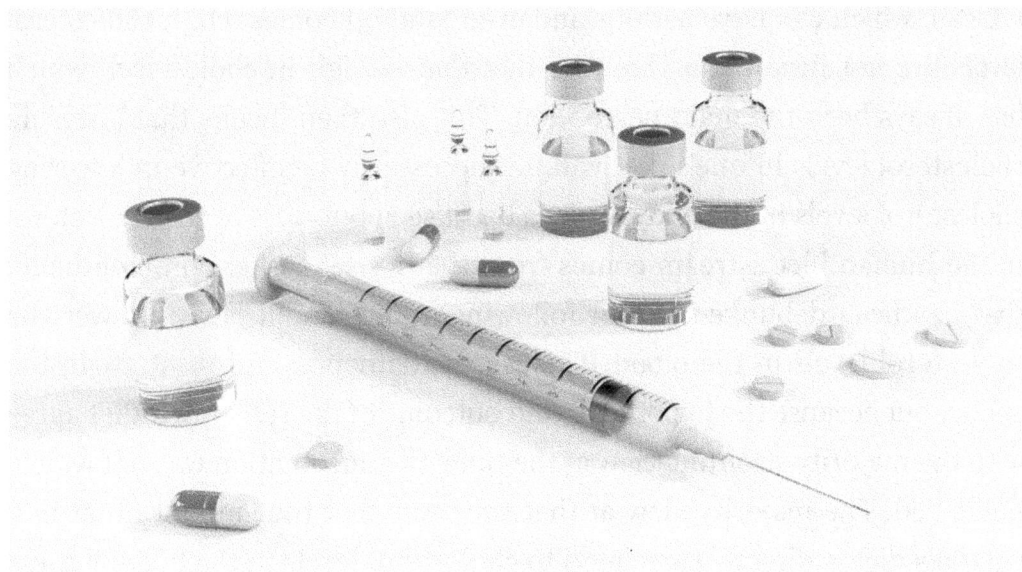

be because our lifestyles are so terribly stressful, and putting food on the table is harder than it used to be? Not that anyone puts food on the table anymore. We all seem to devour it in front of our TV's without checking the calorie density or fat content. One of my favorite comedians says that, if you are even slightly close to being a normal human being, you will stumble into your home, grab the bread from the fridge and eat it by dipping it in anything runnier than bread. There's a lot of truth in that and a good Netflix drama can cause you to eat a lot of food without even noticing, even a whole loaf of bread dipped in anything runnier than bread. So, why do so many people ignore health advice and warnings about high cholesterol? Additionally, is there a way to lower cholesterol that will also address the causes, which are overeating, unhealthy eating, and unmanageable stress levels?

Well, if you decide to follow the 14/10, you can dip your bread in anything runnier than bread during your 10-hour feeding window. However, before you decide to do that straight away, let's look at what an expert, Dr. Jason Fung, says about autophagy and its effects on human cholesterol levels.

High cholesterol is a risk factor for heart disease that can be treated. The cardiovascular diseases that it's a risk factor for includes strokes and heart attacks, which can have serious and even fatal outcomes. High cholesterol levels are not necessarily due to a diet that is high in cholesterol, which has always been the main perception. This also then means that lowering cholesterol levels in one's diet will not necessarily be effective in lowering cholesterol levels in the body. This is because about 80% of the cholesterol in the human bloodstream comes from the liver. Another common belief that has been debunked is that following a diet low in fat will lower the cholesterol levels in the blood. This was actually proven in a study in the 1960s, but because the hypothesis and outcome of the research didn't agree with the majority scientific view at the time, the information was not widely published. The majority view at that time was that the amount of fat in a person's diet is directly correlated to cholesterol levels in the body. I guess it was a case of the minority being regarded as unsubstantial. This changed during the course of time as more studies indicated similar conclusions (Fung, 2016).

When we're talking cholesterol, and you want to get a clear picture of why fasting is effective in maintaining a healthy cholesterol level in the body, there are three friends I'd like you to meet. The first is my bestie and will be your bestie too, HDL. HDL or high-density lipoprotein is the "good choles-terol." Your HDL is a protective friend, so its levels should not be too low, as this can increase the risk of cardiovascular disease. This is why HDL is also known as a "marker of disease" (Fung, 2016).

Next, I want to introduce you to triglycerides. They are also a role-playing component in your cholesterol levels, but you don't want them to visit you in large numbers. In other words, you want low triglyceride levels in your body. An interesting fact about triglycerides is that they are also regarded as disease markers; however, while an HDL imbalance can trigger disease, triglycerides can only be an indication (Fung, 2016).

Finally, I'll introduce you to your least favorable and more slippery friend called LDL or low-density lipoprotein. LDL represents your "bad" choles-terol and should be kept at a low level to maintain optimal health in the human body. Don't let LDL whisper sweet nothings in your ear; you know now that you need to keep this one in check. To make sure that you and LDL have a good understanding, practice regular fasting to show it who's boss (Fung, 2016).

Diabetes

Individuals with type 2 diabetes are not always overweight or obese. We usually associate this condition with being overweight or obese because it is also related to high cholesterol, a bad diet, a sedentary lifestyle, and heart problems. However, let's change the perspective just a little by looking at how fasting combined with a specific eating plan helped type 2 diabetes patients who are not overweight. In other words, the focus was on treating the condition and not added weight loss (Hecht & Scher, 2020).

In this case, the patient was a woman with a BMI of 21.9 in her 50s. A healthy BMI for a woman can be anything between 19 and 25, so her weight would be considered pretty healthy. However, she has been suffering from type 2 diabetes for more than a decade and is unable to control the condition using normal measures that include a diabetic-friendly diet and prescribed medication. The patient had an extremely high blood sugar level of over 9% when she started with the new intermittent fasting plan. Just to provide some context, to be diagnosed with diabetes, your long-term blood sugar levels should be 6,4% or higher. This means that the patient's blood sugar level was up there (Hecht & Scher, 2020).

The patient started with an intervention plan that consisted of an intermittent fasting schedule combined with a ketogenic diet. After four months, her blood-sugar levels dropped to 6.4%, which is the diabetic marker. The prescription medication was then reintroduced and after continuing this routine for the next 14 months, the patient's blood-sugar level dropped below 6%. In this case, the combination of fasting and a ketogenic diet also didn't cause the patient to move under the health BMI levels, so she attained a massive overall health improvement (Hecht & Scher, 2020). If you are suffering from type 2 diabetes and you also need to lose some weight to fall within the healthy BMI range, intermittent fasting as a pathway to autophagy can be just as efficient. We've discussed how beneficial intermittent fasting is for weight loss and fitness, so if your condition requires you to make a lifestyle change, this is definitely a viable option. Always keep in mind that, if you suffer from an illness or health-related condition, the safest option is to discuss a lifestyle change with your physician.

There are also precautions that need to be taken when one decides to start a fasting regime to support type 2 diabetes. First, it is crucial to consult a physician before making any lifestyle changes when suffering from a condition like diabetes. Secondly, a diabetes patient should still give a lot of attention to their diet even if they are fasting. The fasting is not going to cancel out bad dietary choices, and combining the two may even exacerbate the condition. Finally, if you are diabetic and you want to practice fasting, make sure that you don't do extended fasts. Fasting for too long can have an adverse effect on your blood sugar levels if their regulation needs extra care and attention in the first place.

If you want to choose a safe but effective fasting regime, go for a 16/8. If you are not a diabetic, but suffer from insulin resistance, there are studies that indicate that the incorporation of exercise along with fasting can lead to the reversal of this pre-diabetic condition (Autophagy: The Process Changing Our Understanding of Diet and Disease, 2017). This is the cheapest and most effective way to improve your health and improve or even reverse the symptoms and effects of diabetes and insulin resistance.

Cancer

Autophagy can play a role in cancer prevention and cancer treatment. One of the most profound discoveries made by researchers is that, because autophagy promotes the death of cells, it can also be a preventive measure

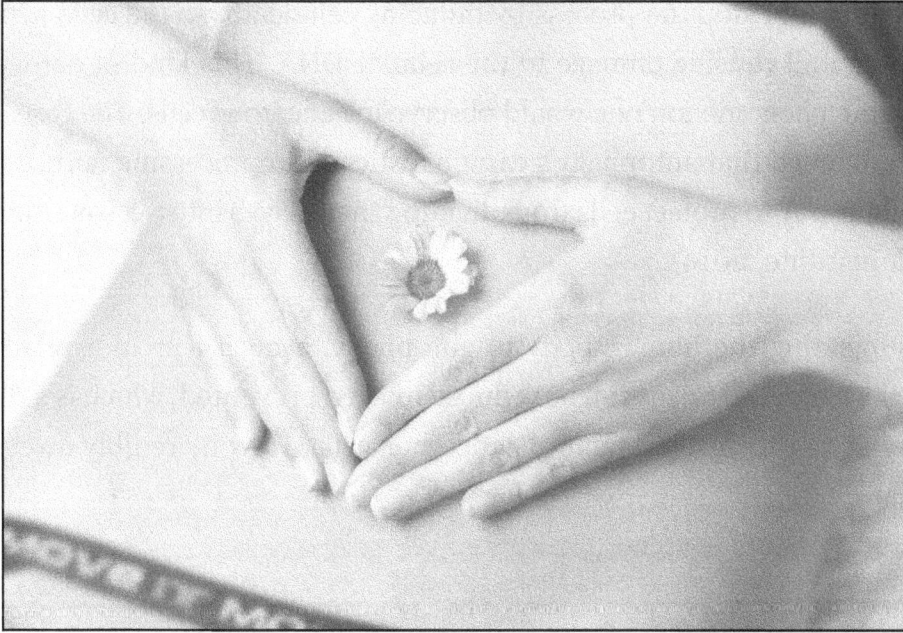

for cancer. This research that was published in the journal *Nature,* goes on to say that autophagy can be described as a "tumor-suppressing pathway" because it acts like a checkpoint that prevents cells from dividing in an uncontrolled nature (Salk Institute, 2019).

The process starts with molecular tips on the end of chromosomes called telomeres that shorten each time a cell divides. The function of telomeres is to protect the end of chromosomes and to prevent them from becoming frazzled due to multiple cell-dividing processes. However, as the telomeres become shorter and shorter, and when they reach a point where they are almost completely gone, the cell enters a crisis situation. During this crisis situation, the unprotected chromosomes can likely fuse and subsequently become dysfunctional, and this is a trademark of some cancer types. What autophagy does in this situation is cause cell death, which means that these dysfunctional cells can no longer divide (Salk Institute, 2019).

To conduct a thorough study on the role of autophagy and cell death in crisis cells, the researchers also took an approach where they allowed cells to divide while observing the systematic shortening of the telomeres until the cells reached the crisis status. This time, autophagy was not used as a mechanism to stop the process by inducing cell death, so the cells kept on dividing and causing damage to the cellular DNA. This kind of damage is the same phenomenon one would observe in cancerous cells. The researchers concluded that autophagy's cannibalistic and reprocessing nature is an excellent way to protect cells from dividing themselves into a crisis situation (Salk Institute, 2019).

By subjecting the human body to autophagy, even if it is in a relatively healthy state, cell crises can be reduced or even prevented, which is a direct pathway to the development of cancerous cells. How incredibly awesome is that?

Alzheimer Disease

Alzheimer disease is known as the cause of advancing dementia that mostly affects the elderly. Alzheimer disease causes a patient to experience advancing, irreversible degenerative cognitive abilities. This neural degradation is caused by multiple pathophysiological processes, which include neuroinflammation, oxidative stress, mitochondrial dysfunction, excitotoxicity, and different types of stress, including proteolytic stress. The aforementioned processes all point to a complex degradation process occurring in the brain, which causes the symptoms of Alzheimer disease. Although extensive research has been conducted on Alzheimer disease, no cure has been found for this debilitating and ultimately fatal condition (Uddin et al., 2018).

Early studies conducted on mice showed that autophagy has the ability to slow down the process of cognitive decline that is associated with Alzheimer disease, and in this study, autophagy was activated in test subjects by applying methods of fasting. This was the first indication that the application of fasting with the aim to activate autophagy can lead to cognitive improvements in patients with Alzheimer disease. Up to this point, pharmaceutical drugs have been used to treat the symptoms of the disease, but no research has ever indicated a mechanism that can trigger a reverse effect or slow down the progression of the disease. Typical behavior associated with an Alzheimer's patient includes difficulty thinking complex and basic thoughts, changes in behavior, and the most common symptom of memory loss. These symptoms are directly related to the degradation of specific areas in the brain, where a dangerous build-up of proteins called plaques collects between nerve cells and proteins called tangles accumulate inside nerve cells. As these plaques and tangles start to spread, they kill vital brain cells the individual needs for optimal cognitive functioning, which causes the degeneration and subsequent disease. For many years, researchers were unable to come up with any indication or hypothesis linked to the cause of this degenerative activity in the brain, but more recent studies have led researchers to believe that it may possibly be linked to not only nutrition, but also the timing of meals (Jorgenson, 2019).

When calorie intake and Alzheimer disease was first linked and researched in tandem, experiments of intermittent fasting were also incorporated to test the effects of meal timing on the condition, development, and possible improvement of Alzheimer disease. This initial research indicated that incorporating fasting periods into the feeding schedules of rats indicated less toxic build-up in the brain and they subsequently had better cognitive function. They also lived longer. As ironic as it sounds, researchers speculate that, by providing your brain with what you would normally see as a starving period of fasting, you would actually be giving your brain the nourishment and maintenance it needs to stay sharp and young. This is because ketones that your body produces after using up its glycogen storage are linked to mental clarity, increased learning, and enhanced memory. Ketones provide the brain with the essential fuel it needs, and some researchers have claimed that ketones can provide the brain with more energy than glycogen. In other words, by constantly eating, we could possibly be starving our brains, and that is why it shows cognitive degeneration at a later stage in life (Jorgenson, 2019).

Currently, studies indicate that intermittent fasting is most likely beneficial for an individual who suffers from Alzheimer disease or has started showing symptoms. However, there is currently a new study being conducted on individuals who are not only Alzheimer patients, but also suffer from obesity and insulin resistance. This is to further investigate the relationship between not only food and Alzheimer disease, but eating habits and elapsed time between meals and how this can be a role-playing factor (Jorgenson, 2019). This most recent study is, at the very least, a strong indication that fasting is already established in these researchers' hypotheses as a role-playing factor when it comes to cognitive health. Consequently, it should also be considered a role-playing factor in the prevention and possible treatment of Alzheimer disease. If autophagy can help individuals to realize early on in their lives that they can minimize their risks of getting Alzheimer disease and be used as a therapeutic tool for those who unfortunately already have the disease, it can make a notable difference in the number of future Alzheimer patients and the declining life quality of current patients.

Heart Failure

There are many different types of heart diseases and dysfunctions one can be diagnosed with and it's frightening to think about. Also, it can happen suddenly with no indication that an individual had any serious health issues. Heart failure is characterized by the heart being unable to pump enough oxygen-rich blood to all the parts of the body. Currently, medical professionals state that there is no cure for heart failure and that more than five million people in the United States suffer from it (Felman, 2018).

Heart failure can occur due to a heart attack, systolic heart failure, or cardiac arrest. These three conditions sound like they can all be part of the same episode, but there are notable differences. A heart attack is characterized by a blockage in a coronary artery that causes damage to the heart muscle. This means that the heart muscle becomes starved of oxygen because blood cannot reach it. In the case of systolic failure, the heart is unable to pump blood to all parts of the body efficiently, so it is actually quite different from a heart attack even though it is also classified as heart failure. Lastly, cardiac arrest occurs when both circulation and the heart stop functioning, which ultimately means that the individual will have no pulse (Felman, 2018).

Some heart failure occurs due to a deteriorated state of autophagy in the body and the fact that it is not as effective as it used to be. The pathological progression that contributes to heart failure is due to the fact that mechanisms that are normally responsible for the reduction of protein are dysfunctional. This means that the maintenance of protein turnover needs to be regulated more strictly to prevent the risk of different forms of heart disease. So, where does autophagy come in? Macroautophagy and chaperone-mediated autophagy (CMA) both help with the transport and reduction or recycling of unwanted protein. The difference between macroautophagy and CMA is that macroautophagy takes big cargo loads while CMA takes smaller loads. Macroautophagy has been studied in research about the loss and gain of heart function, and both approaches indicated the significant role of macroautophagy from a pathological and physiological standpoint.

Fasting, Autophagy, and Mental Health

Mental health plays a pivotal role in our ability to conduct everyday tasks successfully and live a prosperous life. An individual's mental health can also be an indication of whether their physical health needs to be scrutinized and vice versa. Because autophagy can have such transformative effects in the brain and clean out all that neural junk that may cause ill health or cognitive dysfunction, why can't it be likely that this "cleaning-out" can also benefit conditions like depression and anxiety?

Anxiety and depression are sensitive to the stress we experience and whether this stress is acute or chronic. Acute stress is generally seen as healthy stress because the process is not prolonged and the body has the ability to deal with it without much fuss. It can even be used to improve overall health, as in the case of fasting. Chronic stress, however, occurs over an extended period of time and causes feelings of depression and anxiety. This is because the body cannot deal with a stress overload, which leads to negative symptoms. In both of these cases, the hormone cortisol is secreted. Cortisol is also known as the stress hormone and can be either beneficial or toxic, depending on how much of it is being secreted. In acute stress situations, less cortisol is secreted than in chronic stress conditions where a cortisol overload occurs. Unfortunately, chronic stress is more common than we think due to our hectic lifestyles and stressful jobs. The rat race causes our systems to pump out that stress hormone, so we need a way to counter and cope. Exercising is one way to cope with high cortisol levels as it induces autophagy, and by exercising regularly, you can reduce and improve chronic stress levels.

Depression has also been linked to inflammation in the body, and by using intermittent fasting to induce autophagy, it can have a therapeutic effect on inflammation, which can positively influence an individual's depressive state. A fact that is not commonly known regarding the subjects of depression and the treatment of depression is that there is a notable relationship between the brain and the gut. Good gut health is important for good mental health. This is where autophagy plays another pivotal role in reducing depression; it reduces inflammation in the gut by supporting the microbiome, also known as your gut's "ecosystem" (Rose, n.d.).

This interesting relationship between depression, your gut, and your brain is relevant to a balance of different organisms in the gut called dysbiosis, which can affect an individual's mental state, specifically when it comes to depression. If you are aware of such an imbalance, you can treat it effectively with probiotics combined with intermittent fasting. Then, you will know that your gut's sorted (Rose, n.d.).

Chapter 6
Autophagy and Everlasting Youth

If autophagy has been proven to regenerate neural function and play an influential role in disease prevention and the maintenance of health, then it must also have an effect on youthfulness. I mean, if you're healthy and thriving on the inside, then it must show on the outside, and if autophagy can increase your living expectations, then surely, this must show in your exterior aging process. Well, autophagy wouldn't have been such a miracle if it didn't—and it does! There are numerous anti-aging and beauty-related benefits related to the activation of autophagy that range from reversing visible signs of aging to avoiding plastic surgery. In this chapter, we're going to discuss autophagy's anti-aging benefits, what it takes to get you there, and if there are any shortcuts or "autophagy boosters" you need to know about (Ghosh & Pattison, 2018).

Autophagy Is the New Anti-Aging Miracle

Researchers discovered that the cause of aging can be attributed to inflammation in the body. This increasing level of inflammation is hard to counter, and most people try to counter it by taking supplements and topical treatments like collagen or vitamin E-enriched creams for their skin. The supplement aisle at the chemist seems to grow every year and so does the number of health shops. They stay out of the sun, drink their orange juice, eat their fruits and veggies, and jog around the block. Wait! No, that sounds like the 70s. Let's just get back to the present. These days when I walk down the wellness aisle, I see products made from human components that I last learned about in biology class, such as colostrum supplements. Colostrum is a yellowish substance secreted when a mother starts breastfeeding and is also commonly known by health practitioners like nurses and midwives as "liquid gold." I was so surprised to see this on the shelf that I picked it up to see why someone would take it. Apparently, it's a supercharged anti-immune supplement. Who would've thought that this substance could be converted into a supplement? Similarly, when you stroll further down the aisle, you will notice a myriad of different collagen supplements including collagen powder, collagen drinks, collagen protein bars, and collagen shakes and also vitamin E, for that youthful glow. There are even tablets available that induce ketosis in the body for increased fat burning. These supplements can all improve your overall wellbeing and improve the condition of your skin and body. However, how effective are they at reducing that inflammation that is linked to aging? As we know, autophagy works at an intra-cellular level and is quite the process. Can a tablet, a shake, a protein bar, or a cream fix and maintain you from that level? Autophagy truly is an anti-aging miracle.

What do you like most about the figure in the picture on the right? Do you think that the model is an example of conventional beauty? Which physical features do you find most enviable and attractive? If you ask me, I'd say her glowing skin, above all. She also appears to be in good shape, and she

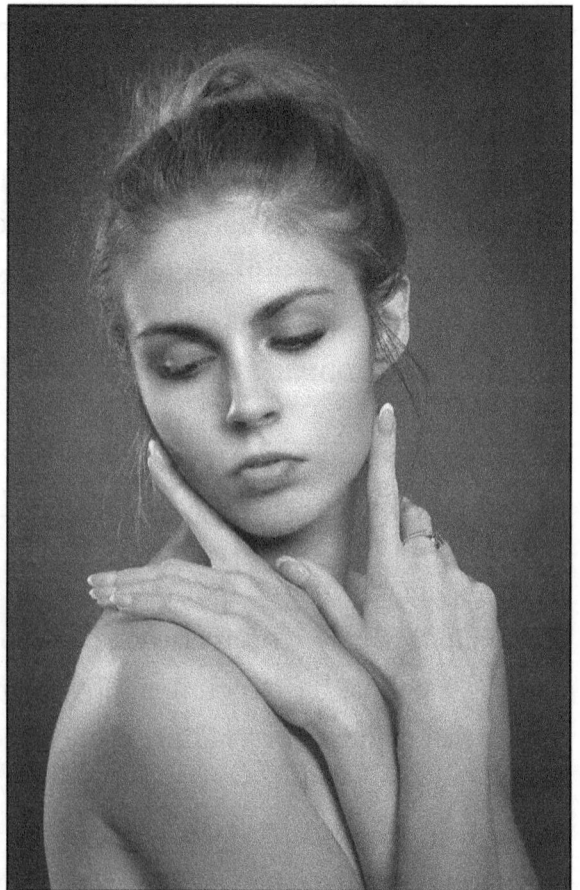

has healthy nails and hair. Do you think she goes for regular treatments to look like this? We may have different opinions about the shape of her ears, nose, and eyes, but one thing we can agree about is that she radiates the kind of youthful health we all want to either achieve or maintain, or both. Autophagy has some beauty tricks up its sleeve.

The Effects of the Citrus Bergamot Fruit

The majority of the world's supply of this magical fruit is found in a rural part of Italy called Calabria known for its beautiful and picturesque land-scapes. Although the Citrus Bergamot is not pleasurable on the palate, it produces an essential oil that has been used in products like Earl Grey tea and cologne for several hundred years. Up until recently, these were the only purposes the Citrus Bergamot was known for until further research was conducted on its incredible effects on human health. It was discovered that the Citrus Bergamot fruit has dynamic effects on aging, health, beauty, and also heart health and cholesterol levels due to unique antioxidant fla-vonoids that can be derived from the fruit. Probably the most profound discovery, made by researchers and experts Naomi Whittel and molecular biologist Dr. Elzbieta Janda, is that the most powerful anti-aging elements lie in the pith of the fruit, which is a part that is generally discarded. The pith contains molecular components that have been shown to dramatically improve and reverse skin damage caused by aging and by assisting skin cells to get rid of the toxins that cause aging. Research has shown that, when the Citrus Bergamot fruit stimulates autophagy in a cell, it influences the cell to undergo a reprogramming process, which can lead to significant anti-aging results. Literally speaking, it reprograms the cell to "act" younger, which means that it will also look younger and be more resilient to age-related complications (Omninutrition, 2019). This is truly a remarkable discovery considering the fact that this fruit has been used for centuries. The Citrus Bergamot fruit is now available in a supplement form and is regarded as one of the most effective foods that can stimulate autophagy on a cellular level.

Autophagy and Healthy Skin

What do we normally do to keep our skin healthy and what are "normal" anti-aging skincare strategies? You know, those secrets passed down from mother to daughter and between sisters that have been secretly sourced from the latest Women's Health magazine's "Beauty" edition? I must admit that I don't even know if that's a thing; I definitely didn't do that growing up with an eccentric mom that didn't really care about skincare, beauty, or makeup. But, my friends and I used to discuss it at length in high school. The staples everyone seems to agree with come down to staying out of the sun or wearing a high SPF sunblock, keeping your skin clean, keeping it moisturized, and following a balanced diet. I do believe in a bi-weekly vitamin C serum or collagen eye cream, but that's definitely not the big-picture anti-aging solution we're all looking for.

Collagen is a protein that is found in abundance in your body when you're young and it has all sorts of functions that include joint support. As you grow older, however, its abundance goes on a sharp decline. Collagen also happens to be the magic ingredient that keeps your skin perky, tight, and hydrated, like a girl's. The way collagen supports the skin can be described like the springs of a mattress. Now, don't think of that old bed that used to stand in the guest room of your grandparent's house; we're talking mattresses with bouncy and perky collagen springs. The cells in the human body that produce collagen are called fibroblasts. Can you see a grand scheme developing yet? These fibroblasts need support as we age so they can stay productive. So, this is the plan:

The lowdown on how to get your youthful complexion back is by activating autophagy and taking the extra measure of consuming a collagen supplement. Activating autophagy will put your fibroblasts into high gear for new collagen production, which will promote hydrated, firm, and perky skin. By adding a regular dose of collagen as a backup, you can ensure that you're getting all the collagen you need. This is where autophagy comes in; it literally improves the production of collagen by stimulating the fibroblasts (Nutrition, 2018).

If you can achieve this, then all those creams and potions will be an added bonus that will bring a glow to your epidermis. Because that may be as deep as skincare creams go. So, that's why you want to stimulate anti-aging from the inside, the natural way. Nature knows best.

Autophagy for a Youthful Body

Another issue that comes along with getting older is loose skin. However, this issue is not exclusively related to aging; individuals who have lost a significant amount of weight can also carry excess skin. The go-to postmodern solution is to go snip-snip. A cosmetic surgeon can remove excess skin from almost anywhere on the body. But what does it cost? Tummy-tucks are extremely common, and these procedures sometimes involve only the removal of excess skin, which means that the procedure was not focused on removing fat from the stomach area. Common areas for older individuals to develop excess skin is in their triceps area, the hips, the neck, chin, and the stomach, although this may be accompanied by belly fat. Using autophagy in the same way you would for creating a youthful complexion is possible if you want to get rid of excess skin; however, there is an upside and a downside. The upside is that it is absolutely free and you may even save some money by buying less food and not paying a cosmetic surgeon. The downside is that the results will not be instantaneous, but it will, in this process, also bring a myriad of other benefits like an unbelievable sense of accomplishment and a bolstered self-esteem.

Other autophagy-related tools you can consider implementing in your lifestyle if you want to get rid of loose skin include polyphenols. Polyphenols are famous for their potent effect on autophagy in the human body. Polyphenols are components found in plants, and their purpose is to protect plants from their environment and the possible harm it may cause to them. This ingredient is almost like the active component in the Citrus Bergamot fruit when you think about the fact that polyphenols are also a plant component assisting your body to activate and reach autophagy. However, polyphenols are specifically beneficial and effective for the health and youth of your skin and can render results for loose skin due to aging or as a result of fat loss or weight loss (Whittel, 2019). From this perspective, you are also using an outside ingredient that is natural to accelerate autophagy in your body and to target a specific area, just as if you decide to use collagen as a supportive supplement to aid the increased fibroblast function you activated through autophagy to achieve a more youthful complexion. If you decide to visit your local health shop in search of polyphenols, you can look out for berberine, resveratrol, and turmeric. Another polyphenol supplement is a tea you can make yourself using the following recipe from autophagy expert Naomi Whittel:

Ingredients:

1 bag of green tea

1 Earl Grey Citrus Bergamot tea bag

1 tablespoon of raw coconut oil

1 Ceylon cinnamon stick

1 optional teaspoon of monk fruit powder

Bring 1 to 1-½ cups of water to the boil in a saucepan or a kettle. After the water has reached the boiling point, pour the water into a large cup or mug, and add the cinnamon and tea bags. Allow the ingredients to steep for at least three minutes or longer if possible. After steeping the ingredients, you can remove the tea bags, add the coconut oil, and stir for about 30 seconds. Naomi's pro-tip is to blend the tea briefly if you want the coconut oil to emulsify and not separate from the rest of the liquid (Whittel, 2018). I guess you can add the monk fruit powder at the initial stage along with the tea bags if you decide to add this optional component.

This recipe, which has also been called "autophagy tea" has optimal benefits as a polyphenol supplement if you drink it first thing in the morning to get your metabolism started and to allow the coconut oil to suppress cravings or an urgency to eat. The ingredients in the tea will also support energy levels during exercise if you choose to make it part of your daily routine and support an extended fat-burning process along with autophagy after you've finished exercising (Whittel, 2018). In addition, looking at the ingredients in this tea, this appears to be a potent autophagy-promoter that, if incorporated with a lifestyle that also supports autophagy-friendly nutrition and eating patterns, can speed up the signs of improved skin-tightening, the reduction of loose or hanging skin, and skin elasticity.

A piece of advice that seems to stick its head out sequentially when reading the advice and opinions of autophagy experts is to make a consistent lifestyle change. This is especially prevalent when you research and educate yourself on the benefits of autophagy in the fields of fitness, weight loss, and beauty. These fields are also the most researched and tried-and-tested areas when it comes to the massive physiological landscape autophagy covers, so giving solid advice can be done without too much doubt and uncertainty. But, the facts and research data are here and it's in black and white. I mean, if you allow autophagy to do its job, wouldn't it just thrive on consuming and repurposing all of the extra skin? I think the real hurdle is, as we mentioned at the beginning of this book, surviving and acclimatizing to the stress you need to expose your body to when you start following a method that will activate autophagy like fasting.

Chapter 7
The Risk Demographic

We have to cover this one before we can go on. There are, in some cases, precautions that need to be taken if an individual has certain relevant age-related or health-related factors that can cause practices like fasting to be harmful. The thing is, before making a major lifestyle change, the smartest step you can take is to visit your physician and discuss it with them. A medical professional, especially one who you have been seeing for an extended period of time, may be able to identify risk factors related to the fasting plan you had in mind, and they can assist you by proposing a modified plan that suits your current health situation or they can give you valuable advice on how to get one started. For example, if you are suffering from insulin resistance and you want to incorporate intermittent fasting to reduce its effects, your doctor can assist by testing your blood sugar levels and referring you to a personal trainer who can help you to safely incorporate exercise into your new routine. This chapter addresses groups of individuals who need to practice caution and who should always consult a medical expert when considering fasting as a means to activating autophagy.

Can Fasting Be Harmful?

Just as there are benefits to fasting, which is regarded as the most efficient way to activate the autophagy mechanism in our bodies, this method should be treated with respect and care because of the stress it puts on the body.

This is why experts recommend a gentle introduction to fasting by fasting for shorter periods in the beginning and not treating feeding windows as an excuse to binge and compensate for the hours spent drinking only water and black coffee. I don't know about you, but I've heard of 14-day water fasts, dry fasts, and other fasting methods that I wouldn't personally recommend because of little scientific backing. Individuals who go on a clean fast for more than 72 hours are known to say that the most profound result is how their hunger disappears completely and their energy levels increase after the first 48 hours. However, when you think about it, introducing food back into your routine before you perish must be pretty tough on the body. How will your digestive system react? Should you start by eating only one stalk of swiss chard? Now that I've successfully planted that scary idea in your head, let's move on to look at legitimate dangerous situations; not because mindful and moderate fasting is dangerous in general, but because in these cases, these individuals have other fish to fry, like having babies, for example.

Fasting and Pregnancy

I think everyone who has been pregnant or who is currently pregnant will definitely understand that this speaks for itself. I don't want to exclude anyone who's never been pregnant or who is not able to become pregnant as I am sure that you can understand this as well. Science has shown us that it's not necessary to "eat for two" as your grandmother would have said, but putting your body into starvation mode, which is literally the opposite, cannot possibly be beneficial for the unborn. However, this discussion will not be completely valid if we don't add the opinions of experts to support my own opinion. The main reason women seem to consider intermittent fasting during pregnancy is for weight maintenance. According to experts, while your adult body may benefit from restricted eating periods, the growing body inside you does not. For a successful pregnancy, the unborn needs nourishment and fuel throughout the day and not just for a few hours, even if you eat all your required calories during those hours. Additionally, there is no supporting evidence that indicates the safety of intermittent fasting during pregnancy, and prolonged fasts cannot possibly be safe or beneficial for such a rapidly growing body. Physicians suggest a moderate calorie

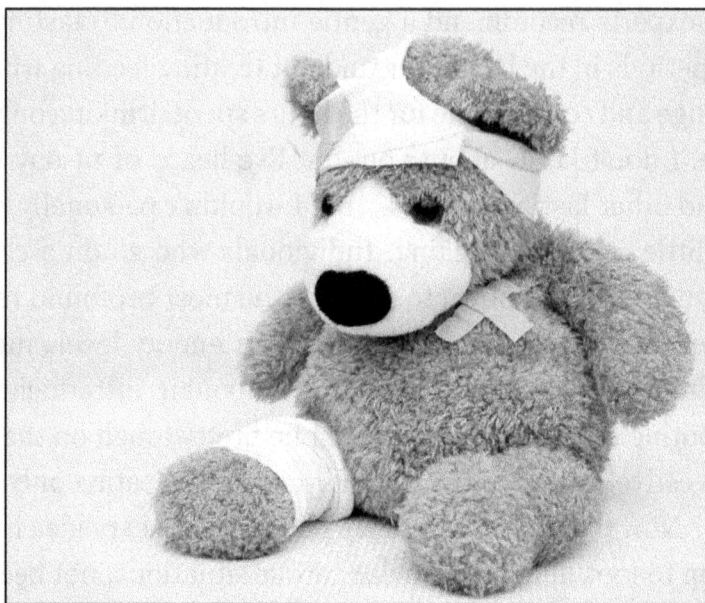

increase, but definitely not to the level where you are eating for two, and instead of pursuing a weight loss strategy like intermittent fasting, weight gain can easily be controlled using other methods like cutting out refined sugar and increasing your level of physical activity. Interestingly enough, medical experts also mention that, when breastfeeding, you may be so hungry that intermittent fasting is not likely to be an option. Using all your food to produce and then provide food? Totally understandable. Finally, trying to actively restrict and time your food intake while also coping with all the changes happening to your body during pregnancy is going to be overwhelming. This is the best time to allow yourself some freedom in order to place as little stress as possible on the unborn. From the experts: After you've given birth and passed the breastfeeding stage, you can gently ease (back) into intermittent fasting to give your metabolism a boost and get your body where you want it to be (Larkin, 2019).

Fasting and Children

Fasting may be introduced to children for religious purposes, which is a completely different discussion, but should you expose a child to intermittent fasting with the aim to activate autophagy for weight loss? Experts in this field say that there are both physiological and psychological pitfalls when applying a fasting strategy to a child's lifestyle. Like an unborn, a child is still in a growing phase and will be rapidly growing until their late teens. Crucial areas of development in a child's anatomy include their cerebrum and muscular structure, and any type of dietary restriction or restricted eating patterns are to be strongly dissuaded. The focus should be on making safe and stable dietary decisions a child can lean on to develop an intact support system for adulthood (Erenzi, 2020). Children have their own unique way of disregarding mealtimes because they "don't feel hungry," but you'll see them making up for it later by eating a triple helping of peanut butter and banana sandwiches. This should in no sense be confused with possible potential for intermittent fasting. Children aren't as concerned about eating and diets as we are except if we imprint that characteristic onto them, so it benefits their physiological development when introducing regular mealtimes. Intense restrictions can have a negative effect on a child's relationship with food, which can cause psychological issues later in life. For example, imagine placing a child on a 16/8 fasting schedule and sending them to school without breakfast, only allowed to drink water because they are too young for black coffee. Or, the child is on a 5:2 fasting schedule, and their fasting days happen to fall over the weekend. They are invited to a birthday party, but they are not allowed to eat a piece of the birthday cake or any of the candy, not even a small piece, because it will break their fast. It does sound preposterous, I know. But that's the lens you have to look through to get the full picture. Imagine how deprived such a child would feel; not only are they deprived of eating a nutritious breakfast that can help them grow a healthy mind and body, but they are also deprived of experiencing the things children do, like going to birthday parties and eating birthday cake. Let's deduce that, due to the nutritional requirements of a growing child and the psychological importance of fitting in among their peers, intermittent fasting should not be something that is forcibly introduced in their lives.

Fasting and Professional Athletes

Many of us don't realize what professional athletes need to do in terms of diet and training to be at the top of their game. There are a lot of different fitness figures and representatives in the industry, but they don't represent the way professional athletes train. They may incorporate some of these athletes' best-kept secrets like carb-cycling and make it accessible to individuals like us who are interested in losing body fat and staying in shape, but it's their job. It has got to be hard to be a top professional athlete, especially on your body, but also on your mind. So, why would professional athletes not be able to benefit from intermittent fasting? Well, firstly, exercise can also activate the autophagy mechanism, and they exercise a lot. The intensity of the exercise a professional athlete does is so much that their body actually works differently from ours. It works on an elevated level, and because of the intensity of their exercise regimes and the timing of their exercise sessions, an intermittent fasting schedule will not work for them. First, if an athlete works out in a fasted state at the level of intensity that is required, their bodies may go so far as to start consuming muscle mass. This is because professional athletes have very little body fat, so it's not like there's an infinite supply of unwanted fat the body can use during autophagy. If this happens, it will only cause the athlete to experience fatigue and physical stress, which are conditions they work extremely hard to avoid. Let's take this to a practical level by looking at the training regime and dietary requirements of Olympic swimmer, Michael Phelps. Michael Phelps is the perfect example of how to cram a seemingly-impossible number of calories into a human body while doing a seemingly-impossible amount of exercise. While exercising 25 to 30 hours a week, he also consumes 12,000 calories a day. Yes, I'm serious. Let's start by looking at his training schedule. His training can be divided into three sets of swimming exercises all with the aim of developing a different technique, and then there is also a pretty tough weightlifting program he follows twice a week. The first two swimming training sessions are meant to develop and maintain the different styles, and the third is for speed and endurance. The additional strength training, which is a combination of dumbbell and compound exercises, is to support endurance in the water (Ellis, 2020).

Apart from Phelps' favorite cereal being Cinnamon Toast Crunch, he also eats a wide variety of other high-calorie foods—you know, the kind of foods we normally avoid, weigh, or binge on in secret. Here's the lowdown: His meals generally come in at about 4,000 calories each. For breakfast, he eats the kind of egg sandwich I would eat if I had a massive hangover. Actually, he eats three of them. They contain fried eggs, cheese, tomato, mayonnaise, fried onions, and lettuce. After this, he then drinks two cups of coffee, eats an omelet made from five eggs, more eggs in his three slices of French toast, three chocolate-chip pancakes, and a slightly out-of-place bowl of grits. When lunch comes around, he proceeds to eat two sizable ham and mayonnaise sandwiches and a pound of pasta. Just in case the calories don't add up, he adds another 1,000 calories' worth of energy drinks. When dinner rolls around, he eats another pound of pasta and a whole pizza and washes it down with another 1,000 calories' worth of energy drinks. Between these meals, he trains intensively for five to six hours a day (RichieMuscleProdigy, 2011).

Considering everything you just had to absorb about this massive diet and strenuous exercise regime, you can probably understand that an athlete like Michael Phelps is not going to experience a pleasant feeling in his gut if he eats a combo-meal before a training session, like lunch and breakfast together. Intermittent fasting's main requirement is that you consume all of your calories within a specific feeding window, which makes it really ineffective for professional athletes because they need to consume, on average, 3,000 calories per day, and in Phelps' case a whopping 12,000. Imagine having to eat all of those calories in the span of eight hours and combine it with intense training sessions. Three thousand calories equals six Big Macs or three pints of Ben & Jerry's. Twelve thousand calories equals 24 Big Macs or 12 pints of Ben & Jerry's. Imagine the intestinal confusion, trauma, and subsequent cramps. It'd put me off intermittent fasting for life. Although, I think if someone were to force-feed me six Big Macs or three pints of Ben & Jerry's, I'd also avoid these outlets for the rest of my life. The bottom line here is that professional athletes keep their bodies clean on the inside by doing what they do. They have to live a healthy lifestyle to perform their best, and with this, I mean consuming nutrient-rich foods and maintaining a very low body fat percentage. Taking extra measures to maintain the levels of fat in their body may not be the best idea. We learned earlier that exercise can also activate autophagy in the body, and if you take it to their level, then why add fasting? (Calvert, 2012).

Fasting and Eating Disorders

An eating disorder that specialists have claimed to be dangerously similar to intermittent fasting is anorexia nervosa. Not because intermittent fasting is in itself a disorder or toxic, but because these similarities, which include abstaining from eating for specific periods of times, may lead individuals who suffer from anorexia nervosa to misuse the basic concepts of intermittent fasting or prolonged fasting to exacerbate their illness. About 14% of Americans have admitted that they use intermittent fasting for the sole reason of losing weight. The number of these individuals who suffer from anorexia nervosa is not currently known, but they will be using the fasting method in a compulsive manner in order to drop pounds that they cannot afford to lose (Fredricks, n.d.).

Anorexia Nervosa is a condition that can develop during childhood and is more common among females than males. However, the diagnostic numbers for boys has been increasing in recent years. The statistics on this condition indicates that it is about as common as autism. There are several ways in which one can identify anorexic behavior, and these diagnostic signs are also used by medical professionals to identify and diagnose an individual with anorexia nervosa. The first indication is that of an individual who conducts self-imposed weight loss by means of extreme calorie restriction through dieting, vomiting, or other restrictive measures that leads to a BMI of less than 17.5. Looking back at what was said of healthy BMIs for women, the lowest level an individual's BMI can be on before officially being classified as underweight is between 18 and 19. The second indication is that the individual shows a peculiar attitude towards body weight and food. There is usually an intense preoccupation with losing weight and being thinner even if the individual's BMI is below normal. Although the BMI indicates they are underweight, they still feel overweight and fat. They experience an undisguised fear of gaining weight and are also persistently busy interfering with any factors that could cause this to happen. Someone who suffers from anorexia will, for example, do everything in their power to avoid a situation where they will be expected to eat what they consider to be "too many calories." Also, if they land in such a situation, they will eat the absolute minimum and most likely would've already planned an escape route in their heads for where they can get rid of the food. For example, they will identify the bathroom at the lonely end of the hallway upstairs, where they can go to purge themselves of any unnecessary calories if they were to be put in a position to consume them. This bathroom is better than the one downstairs, where someone might hear what's going on. The consumption of unplanned or unwanted calories causes anorexia patients a lot of anxiety, and that is why they use intervention techniques like vomiting. The final indication may be that the individual is no longer having her period regularly, but this is only a viable sign if she is not on contraceptives (Fredricks, n.d.).

For someone who suffers from anorexia, fasting must seem like the ultimate weight-control tool that will ensure they don't gain weight or experience any issues when confronted with food. The problem is that they cannot differentiate between healthy fasting and starvation because of their warped view on food and weight loss in the first place. When you implement intermittent fasting in your lifestyle, you see food as an essential tool for nourishment and if you are a healthy individual, from a psychological perspective, intermittent fasting can most likely improve your relationship with food. However, anorectics , who often suffer from body dysmorphic disorder and are not able to see their bodies as we see them, will abuse fasting and use it to try and eliminate calorie intake as much as possible. They will always see someone bigger and fatter in the mirror, and they will hate themselves for it and keep on pushing even harder to get rid of the imperfections they see. This is an extremely sad situation as an anorectic will start by implementing what they perceive to be intermittent fasting, but what they are actually doing is engaging in restricted eating and starving, which causes their body to develop nutritional deficiencies and become malnourished. If fasting turns into starvation and it goes too far, the body can start metabolizing essential tissues that even include heart tissue. When the body starts doing this, it's a sure-fire sign that starvation is occurring and not healthy fasting (Fredricks, n.d.).

It is possible that, if someone is diagnosed with anorexia nervosa, they won't be able to make the choice to avoid intermittent fasting for themselves as a different reality is playing in their minds. If you know of someone who wants to try intermittent fasting for weight loss reasons, but they actually appear to be underweight and obsessed with dieting, binging, and purging, exercising excessively in relation to their dietary intake or BMI, or taking laxatives too often without consulting a doctor, they may need the help of a psychologist. All the behaviors mentioned above can be observed as obsessive-compulsive patterns in anorectic patients, and these individuals have a high likelihood of exhibiting suicidal behavior. Their warped approach to intermittent fasting can cause their bodies many health issues, and if they don't seek treatment for their psychological state, they may become seriously ill (Fredricks, n.d.).

Fasting for Men Versus Fasting for Women

So, no-one's saying that men are better than women or vice versa. But because we are looking at all the facets of autophagy and how to induce it using intermittent fasting, an important focal point has to be the differences between the male and female body, their unique physiological functions, and how different types of fasting schedules can impact them. I suspect that these fundamental differences in our physiological processing and makeup also goes back to that same evolutionary theory the source of autophagy is also theorized to have come from many, many moons ago. So, let's look at some biological differences between men and women and how this can affect their intermittent fasting choices and habits.

Specific fasting schedules, like alternate day fasting, was used in a study that included non-obese men and women. According to this study, men and women's insulin sensitivity was affected differently by alternate day fasting. In the case of men, it had a positive effect by improving their insulin sensitivity when they reached their feeding window or next meal. However, women's insulin sensitivity worsened on this schedule due to a declined glucose clearance. These different reactions show that there is actually a difference in the way men and women regulate blood sugar. Although no hypotheses have yet to be proven, theories include the fact that men and women have differences in their body composition and women seem to have a different way of metabolizing carbohydrates. On top of this, studies indicate that the livers of men and women don't function in exactly the same way in a fasted state. This means that glucose regulation is going to be different in a man's body while fasting because women release less glucagon than men during a fasted state (Nutrafol Team, 2019). If I remember correctly, glucagon is a hormone that the liver secretes to stabilize blood sugar when we are in a fasted state or during exercise. Now, I wonder why a woman's body would do this. Do you think that, perhaps, a woman's body has a natural mechanism to prevent her from fasting for too long? If the liver doesn't secrete as much glucagon, she will probably feel like eating something. A woman should naturally have more body fat than a man, so could the liver possibly be counteracting a woman's attempt to lose too much body fat by secreting less glucagon? This is my ten cents, of course, but I find the concept fascinating. If a woman loses too much body fat, she experiences hormonal issues and can consequently lose her fertility status and her ability to have children, which is not what Mother Nature wants from an evolutionary perspective. A man, on the other hand, can survive with a significantly lower body fat percentage.

While we're on the subject of fertility and female body fat percentage, you may be interested to know that a study conducted on young female rats showed that a restricted diet and fasting regime affected their fertility. There is a reason for women to be more gentle on themselves when they start a fasting regime because, even though some women have claimed intermittent fasting to be life-changing and wildly successful, other women have reported symptoms such as metabolic issues, losing their periods completely, binge-eating episodes, and even early-onset menopause, and we're talking about women as young as in their early twenties (Kollias, 2015). This is a clear indication that, as a woman, you need to be more compassionate with yourself if you decide to incorporate fasting into your life. We appear to have more diversity when it comes to hormone levels than men, so there is no one size fits all fasting formula for women. Even if you decide to incorporate a 14/10 and make slight dietary changes, talk to your doctor first. It's not that you can't do it at all; I mean, we've talked about many benefits and success stories so far that include women. However, because women are special and important to nature and their bodily health has different requirements, extra precautions should be taken. Do what feels good for you. Feeling a bit hungry, for example, is not necessarily a life-threatening symptom or one that will have serious health consequences, but there are others you can look out for like metabolic and fertility issues.

Hopefully, this chapter made you aware of the fact that fasting should sometimes be avoided completely and at other times be approached with caution. By looking at the facts and studies, a fasting regime or schedule can be life-threatening to someone with poor mental health just because of the behavior it encourages. Additionally, it can be misunderstood as a way to maintain weight or to even lose weight while you have another life growing inside you. When planning or investigating a fasting schedule that will work for you, these details should be in the back of your mind. When your friends and family indicate some of these risky behaviors, you will be aware of them and you can encourage them to see a health professional. As well, if you are a woman and fasting just doesn't feel right for you or if it makes you feel downright unhealthy, you will be forearmed with a general idea of what this type of eating plan can potentially do to your hormones or to your relationship with food.

Chapter 8
Find Your Niche

Now, after reading information that began with the sciency definitions of the different types of autophagy, proceeded through the different methods of fasting and exercise strategies, and ended with risk demographics, where do you begin your own journey? There have been tips and hacks mentioned along the way, but this chapter is dedicated to providing a step-by-step guide that can help you assess where you are mentally and physically and how this will translate to the best lifestyle choices for you. When we make lifestyle choices, we want them to have lasting effects, especially if the effects are as promising as those mentioned in this book. Let's finish off by taking a mindful journey of introspection and, in this process, give all of this information a personal meaning and purpose.

Being Mindful About Your Needs

We have dreams, aspirations, wants, and needs. Which comes first and what does it mean to be mindful? Mindfulness is the act of looking at yourself and your environment in a gentle and caring way. This involves being aware of your existence, awareness, and thoughts, how your body feels, and how you feel in your environment (*Mindfulness Definition | What Is Mindfulness*, 2019). Now, take this approach and focus it on your body image, physical needs, and your mental needs. How healthy is your body? Do you feel comfortable in your body? If your answer is no, can you explain why not?

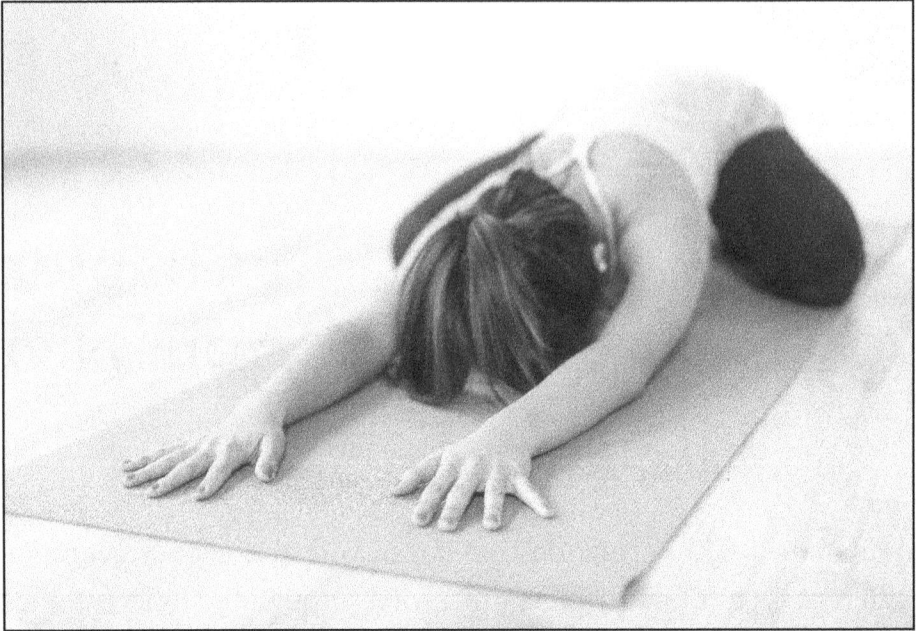

Is it the way your body looks or how it feels on the inside that bothers you? Inspecting your true feelings about your body image may provide an indication of how you will handle intermittent fasting mentally and if it can possibly improve your relationship with food. For example, we discussed earlier that some women reported episodes of binging after trying intermittent fasting. How would you explain this behavior if someone asked you your opinion about it? Do you think it could be a mental or physiological response to fasting? Or is it a hunger thing? If you get in touch with your body mindfully, you can determine how you will respond to fasting psychologically and if it will make you a healthier person mentally. We know that it can provide mental clarity and focus, but if you can identify the exact reasons why you want to start intermittent fasting by sitting or lying down, relaxing, and sinking deeply into your mind, you will be off to a healthy and realistic start. You can practice mindful meditation by visualizing your goal. What is it that you want clarity about? Create a space for yourself where there are minimal disruptions and where you can quietly relax and think. Sitting or lying down, get in touch with your body just as deeply as autophagy works to heal your body. Most of us know why we want to do something, but if it involves a lifestyle choice or a similar major change, thinking about it deeply may reveal the true feelings. The reason why I'm suggesting this is because I tend to do the opposite; I tend to go through multiple phases of trial and error in true drama queen style before I realize that I made a complete fool of myself by involving everyone, including the neighbor's cat. So, this suggestion is offered with love and has also been extensively researched and proven to be very effective. It has even been suggested to me by a few hesitant bystanders. "Know thyself," they say.

Assessing Your Lifestyle and Habits

Another important point you can use when referring to all the facts and advice in this book is where you're at physically and how you prefer to live your life. This is important because if the fasting method you choose to follow doesn't fit into your current lifestyle, it's not likely to stick, except if you need to make a drastic change for the sake of your health. If you're a social butterfly who likes their nights out every now and then, you still have several options. You can do a 5:2 or a 6:1 and just make sure that your fasting window doesn't fall over the weekend or whenever you're likely to go out. However, this doesn't mean that you won't have that one day when you are meant to be fasting and someone invites you out for a glass of wine or a gin and tonic. Be flexible with yourself and know that cheating one time won't crash your whole routine, so you can plan to fast the next day or be okay with breaking your fast once in a while. However, if you like going out at night to party, then following an eating schedule according to your circadian rhythm is definitely not going to work for you. You'll be sitting at the bar sipping sparkling water all night.

Something that I find plays a significant role in successful intermittent fasting is a person's level of perfectionism. There are going to be those odd days when you can't stick to your fasting window 100%, and this can drive some people up the wall, especially when they know the physiological process that happens every time they fast and why it's important to restrict calorie intake. By the way, I'm not talking to the dirty fasters. I don't think an extreme perfectionist will be able to mentally cope with a dirty fast; one has to be a bit more relaxed for that. The moral of this jibber-jabber is *don't be too hard on yourself*. You will find a fasting routine that is the most compatible with your lifestyle, but you will also have those days when it's impossible to fast because other people are making too many of your decisions. Of course, as long as you maintain the duration of the fasting and feeding windows, you can determine their times.

Moving on to physical fitness and whether you have fitness goals, you can start by looking at your current fitness level. In Chapter 4, there are several guidelines on how you can incorporate fasted exercise for different fitness levels, but you don't have to stick to HIIT and WIRT. These are recommendations for the most efficient fat loss or muscle building. But, what if you want to have some fun, and you don't think burpees are fun? I love doing yoga and dancing workouts, especially those where I go all wild and act like an imbecile for 45 minutes. I always make sure that the curtains are closed, but I blast the music at a level that rattles the grotesque china I inherited from my grandmother. That makes fasted exercise worth it for me. I'm also sure to include some high intensity exercise in there somewhere, maybe just not in timed intervals. If you are a newbie to working out, then it's even more beneficial to do a workout that you enjoy. You will feel great after any workout, and that's why HIIT is so popular. You will really feel like the king or queen of the jungle. You can't climb a flight of stairs by jumping from the bottom to the top, so start where you're comfortable, push yourself a little, and make it fun and effective by keeping your goal in mind as well as what the experts say.

What's for Dinner? Is There Dinner?

The question of what to eat when fasting is probably where you are going to get the most diverse and even opposing opinions. Even though we spoke about this a bit in Chapter 2, you'll benefit from digging deeper and exploring your dietary wants and needs. Again, doing it mindfully will bring you the best results. The word you'll hear most often is "Keto." The Keto (keto-genic) diet's purpose is to put your body in ketosis, which is something that will happen when you fast. So, you have to ask yourself if these dietary restrictions are necessary for everyone. In the case of the patient who strug-gled with type 2 diabetes and couldn't find any other successful treatment, the combination of intermittent fasting and Keto was very successful. How does your health compare to that patient's? Can you make more modest modifications to your diet like cutting out refined carbs and sugar to reach your health goals?

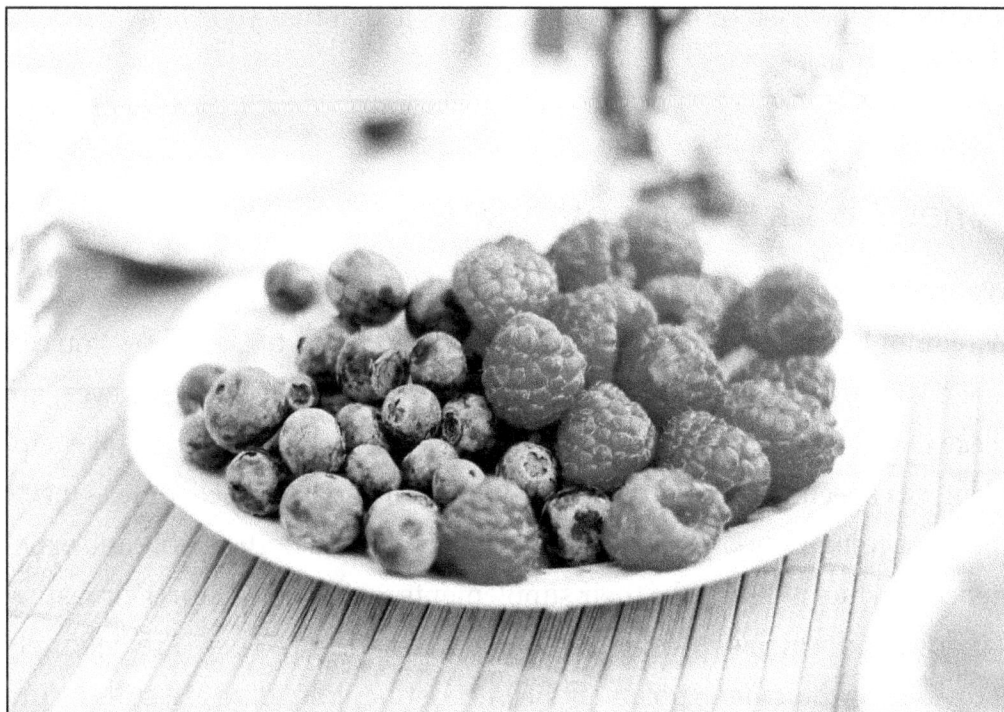

One of the concepts that intermittent fasting apps and programs so often subscribe to is that you can still eat what you want and as much as you want. It's fine to use this advertising strategy for someone who doesn't binge or overeat constantly, but is it productive to market intermittent fasting in this way? If I could make an educated guess, I'd assume that the ratio-nale behind this slogan is that the fasting practice will automatically cure whatever eating problem the individual had when they started; possibly by shrinking their stomach or by regulating the secretion of ghrelin and leptin. However, I don't think this is the way fasting should be approached if you want to get the most out of it; and you can really get a lot out of it. When you decide to include intermittent fasting in your lifestyle and you look at your eating habits and diet, the best way to go is to follow a nutrient-dense diet. If you do want to make any major dietary changes, your best bet is to see a nutritionist or a doctor first. When it comes to which diet to follow, people's dietary needs and lifestyles are too diverse to be able to say one specific diet is your best bet, especially if the diet is very restrictive. For yourself, be honest about what your body needs and how much it needs, and remember that feeling peckish or hungry is not always a sign that your body needs to consume calories.

What About Supplements?

We spoke about foods that activate and accelerate autophagy like the Citrus Bergamot Fruit, other foods like cinnamon and green tea, and how you can make your own autophagy tea using a superpowered recipe. However, are these the same as supplements for autophagy, and do you need to take supplements specifically because you are following a fasting schedule? One of the most commonly-asked questions on the web from both newbie and experienced fasters is "Can take their supplements while they are in their fasting window, and which supplements are most beneficial?" There are definitely individuals who take supplements while fasting, but some are still unsure about the timing and the types. Foods that accelerate autophagy also have health benefits, but they are not necessarily categorized as supplements; maybe because when you think about supplements, you think tablets and powders. One of the reasons you might consider taking extra supplements when fasting is if you combine fasting with regular exercise and you don't have the time to consistently prepare nutrient-dense meals. So, supplements should not really be seen as a fasting prerequisite, but as a helping hand if you need nutritional support. Apart from taking your multivitamin daily, you can consider these supplements and vitamins as an add-on for optimal fasting health.

The best way to support your body while following a fasting schedule is to eat the most nutritious foods available to you. However, if you are one who loves to spend time making delicious, nutrient-dense meals, but ends up occasionally buying ready-to-eat ones, you may want to consider taking some extra supplements. There are three supplements suggested specifically for a fasting lifestyle due to their targeted effect on different areas of the body. Firstly, one you can check out is your vitamin D level. It's as easy as spending half an hour in the sun every day to fix, but some individuals can have a more serious deficiency, and vitamin D is important for optimal immune function. If you suspect a vitamin D deficiency, you can consult your doctor and go for a blood test, which will give you the confirmation you need. Fasting is also targeted at activating autophagy, which strengthens the immune system, so by filling a small gap by supplementing vitamin D, you can reach the health levels you've been aspiring to.

Next, you can look at your magnesium intake. This mineral has many benefits that can make your fasting experience much easier and, dare I say, potentially less painful. If you are very active while fasting, adding magnesium will deal with your muscle cramps decisively in a non-nonsense and hands-on manner. It is furthermore essential, not only for sleeping well but also to deter that overwhelming sensation of fatigue. It's like a double-sided coin; a decent magnesium intake will ensure that your nervous system and muscle control are regulated at all times.

Finally, one that not only intermittent fasters, but most individuals, can consider coveting is a decent Omega-3 fatty acid support supplement. These essential fats are not made by the body itself, so it needs to be ingested regularly. It is crucial for healthy brain function, eye function, immune health, and heart health. You can't lose with a good Omega-3 supplement, especially if you are fasting regularly (Shah, 2020).

Now, the timing of supplement intake is also a confusing topic because some say that supplements will activate insulin secretion and break your fast, and others say they won't. If you are a dirty faster, this shouldn't be an issue, except if your supplements should be taken with a meal. For intermittent fasters who want to keep their fasting windows clean to heighten their chances of activating autophagy, professionals suggest that you take supplements in your feeding window. First, because then there is no way that it can possibly break your fast. Second, it can improve the absorption of the supplement you are taking (Shah, 2020).

Because we all have different nutritional needs, just like we will not likely all be compatible with the same fasting schedule and lifestyle, it's best to check with your doctor for nutritional deficiencies and for supplements prescribed specifically for these issues. Getting these nutrients through dietary intake is ideal, so make sure that you use supplements only if you are not able to get the nutrients through your diet.

Conclusion

Before I go, I need to tell you a story. It's my own story about how I experienced intermittent fasting and how I developed my ideal rhythm. Boy, was it hard! Not only because I was hungry, but because I live with a partner who thinks intermittent fasting is a complete farce. I decided to give intermittent fasting a try because I used to have a job where I was active all day, always busy doing something, and always under an immense amount of stress. Although my eating habits were something out of a dietary horror film, I was in good shape because I was so active all day. I was also still in my late 20s, so I think I had youthful metabolism to carry me through all the sugar I consumed. I would eat two slabs of chocolate and a giant muffin before work, drink coffee with a lot of sugar during the day, and go home to eat a massive, carby dinner and some more bedtime candy. However, my working situation changed as I relocated with my partner, and although my activity levels went way down, my sugar intake didn't. I generally didn't feel very well and fell into a depression. I didn't want to feel that way, but a change seemed like a mountain to climb at that point. So, that is how my journey started.

I made a lot of mistakes in the beginning. The first mistake I made was the ultimate rookie mistake; I thought that I will just magically be able to not eat for an extended period of time. So, I started with the 16/8. Now, we now know that you can arrange the 16/8 any way you want, but the way that worked for me and for my partner was if I skipped breakfast. This was because we had a dinner thing; we would prepare and eat dinner together.

My habits did not let me succeed though. Breakfast is my favorite meal of the day. When I wake up, I can't wait to eat breakfast. While I waited for the coffee on the stove, I took bites of my partner's cereal because I didn't want to start eating mine until I was back in bed. I thought that he was not going to notice; I poured in some extra cereal just to make sure that there would still be enough left when the bowl finally reached him. I know, I'm terrible. He didn't even know I did this. At other times, I would eat another bowl of cereal or a peanut butter sandwich an hour later for a second breakfast, but by then, he would be off to work. The reason I'm spilling my guts about my naughty breakfast routine is just to tell you how much I like breakfast, and I am absolutely ravenous in the morning. Drinking black coffee instead of two sugars was actually not so bad, and it stuck. However, I was only able to do the 16/8 for two days, and I would sit looking at my watch from 11:00 to 12:00, waiting for lunch. That obviously didn't work for me.

So, I had to go back to the drawing board. I know that I am less hungry in the evening and that it would be easier for me to fast that way around, but it didn't feel right to change a habit that had been a part of our relationship for more than seven years. It's that classic "how are you going to fit intermittent fasting into a lifestyle you share with someone?" dilemma. So, I went and watched a ton of online videos and did some reading. I then decided to start the 14/10, which would also extend my breakfast until at least 9:00. Along with this decision, I decided to suck it up and to stop eating my partner's cereal secretly. So, my morning began with a black coffee, and I made him cereal and coffee like I always did. No secret bites. This gradually morphed into a habit, although I asked my partner to meet me halfway by us making dinner a bit earlier in the evening so that I don't have to wait so long to eat breakfast. This helped. However, after a few weeks, I noticed that I was not constantly watching the time on my Fitbit, waiting for the moment I could start eating because I didn't constantly feel hungry. My obsession with the timing of feeding and fasting windows had also disappeared. The mental obstacle was the biggest and hardest to overcome.

I also exercised regularly, but it used to be mainly low-intensity exercise like walking. So, I decided to step it up a notch and combine it with high-intensity exercise three times a week. I was able to do this with a workout partner, which made it a lot easier. The only thing left for me to do was to stop eating too much candy, which was one of the reasons I decided to start fasting in the first place. For me, it was about waking my body up to its natural eating rhythm, nutritional requirements, making it less dependent on sugar. It worked. Once I decided to be less forceful, I glided into the pattern and started to feel what my body needed. My need for sugar gradually declined, but I also learned that I shouldn't go shopping for food on a completely empty stomach or I might just buy a mound of Twinkies. So, I'd have a cup of black coffee if I was fasting or a small snack during my feeding window before I entered any shop.

Although I lost weight, the most profound difference for me was my mental state. I believe it was because of the mind shift that I started losing weight. At the beginning of my fasting journey, I visited my doctor, who conducted a full blood test. There were no issues, but she did warn me not to be too obsessive about the whole process. I think that this is a mistake many people make because, due to the hype and claims circulating about autophagy and fasting, they expect to see immediate results. However, although autophagy is extremely effective and a natural process, you need to give your body time to adapt and thrive. Impatience and forcefulness will add extra stress, which is, ironically, going to slow down the process.

The purpose of this intermittent fasting guide is to give you a multifaceted idea of what autophagy is, how intermittent fasting ties to the process of autophagy, and in how many different ways it can be implemented or used to activate autophagy. It is a clear illustration of how intelligent the human body really is and how this intelligence lay hidden for so long until it was rediscovered half a century ago. Now, it is one of the most popular research topics in healthcare due to its diverse healing and preventive qualities.

You have read an almost immeasurable amount of information; from the cellular process, to the fasting schedules, the implementation of exercise, and how autophagy can be of benefit while aging. This is factual information you can use in your fasting journey. Also, make sure to take note of the risk demographic and consult a doctor if you want to make a lifestyle change. Finally, I hope that my story can help you to avoid some mistakes or provide you with some good ideas for your own fasting journey. A good start is to refrain from eating your partner's cereal behind their back!

May you have a prosperous and healthy fasting experience that will give you the results you strive for.

References

Ashford, T. P., & Porter, K. R. (1962). CYTOPLASMIC COMPONENTS IN
HEPATIC CELL LYSOSOMES. *The Journal of Cell Biology, 12*(1), 198–202.
https://doi.org/10.1083/jcb.12.1.198

Autophagy: the process changing our understanding of diet and disease.
(2017, October 11). Diabetes. https://www.diabetes.co.uk/blog/2017/10/
autophagy-process-changing-understanding-diet-disease/

Badadani, M. (2012, September 6). *Autophagy Mechanism, Regulation,
Functions, and Disorders.* ISRN Cell Biology. https://www.hindawi.com/
journals/isrn/2012/927064/

Beaver, M. (2019, February 28). *Dirty Fasting. What It Is And How It Can Affect
Your Weight Loss.* Practically Perfect Meg. https://www.practicallyperfectmeg.
com/home/dirtyfasting

Bjarnadottir, A., Kubala, J., & Tinsley, G. (2020, August 4). *Alternate-
Day Fasting.* Healthline. https://www.healthline.com/nutrition/
alternate-day-fasting-guide#1

Calvert, M. (2012, December 18). *Why Intermittent Fasting Is Unsuitable for
Athletes.* STACK. https://www.stack.com/a/intermittent-fasting

Coulson, C. (2020, June 7). *Stages of Fasting - What Happens When
You Fast?* 7Sigma Physiques. https://7sigmaphysiques.com/
stages-of-fasting-what-happens-when-you-fast/

de Cabo, R., & Mattson, M. P. (2019). Effects of Intermittent Fasting on Health, Aging, and Disease. *New England Journal of Medicine, 381*(26), 2541–2551. https://doi.org/10.1056/nejmra1905136

Ellis, N. (2020, April 3). *Michael Phelps Workout, Daily Routine and Diet - Stunning Facts*. The Fitness Folder. https://thefitnessfolder.com/michael-phelps-workout-routine-diet

Erenzi. (2020, January 21). *Is Intermittent Fasting Safe For My Child?* Children's Health – Every Kid Counts. https://blog.gachildrens.org/2020/01/21/is-intermittent-fasting-safe-for-my-child/

Felman, A. (2018, February 17). *Heart disease: Types, causes, and treatments* (D. Sullivan (Ed.)). Www.Medicalnewstoday.Com. https://www.medicalnewstoday.com/articles/237191

Fredricks, R. (n.d.). *Anorexia Nervosa and Fasting - Eating Disorders (Anorexia, Bulimia, Binge Eating) Professional Treatment, & Help*. MentalHelp.Net. https://www.mentalhelp.net/blogs/anorexia-nervosa-and-fasting/

Fung, J. (2016a, October 5). *How to Renew Your Body: Fasting and Autophagy*. Diet Doctor. https://www.dietdoctor.com/renew-body-fasting-autophagy

Fung, J. (2016b, November 6). *Fasting and cholesterol*. Diet Doctor. https://www.dietdoctor.com/fasting-and-cholesterol

Fung, J. (2018, November 25). *Diet Doctor*. Diet Doctor. https://www.dietdoctor.com/does-fasting-burn-muscle

Fung, J., & Scher, B. (2020, July 18). *Intermittent Fasting for Beginners*. Diet Doctor. https://www.dietdoctor.com/intermittent-fasting#:~:text=20%3A4

Ghosh, R., & Pattison, J. S. (2018, January 18). *Macroautophagy and Chaperone-Mediated Autophagy in Heart Failure: The Known and the Unknown*. Oxidative Medicine and Cellular Longevity. https://www.hindawi.com/journals/omcl/2018/8602041/

Hecht, A., & Scher, B. (2020, July 18). *Reverse Type 2 Diabetes with Fasting and Keto, Without Losing Weight*. Diet Doctor. https://www.dietdoctor.com/reverse-type-2-diabetes-with-fasting-and-keto-without-losing-weight

Intermittent Fasting 101 — The Ultimate Beginner's Guide. (2020, April 21). Healthline. https://www.healthline.com/nutrition/intermittent-fasting-guide#1

Jarreau, P. (2019, February 26). *The 5 Stages of Intermittent Fasting*. LIFE Apps | LIVE and LEARN. https://lifeapps.io/fasting/the-5-stages-of-intermittent-fasting/

Jockers, D. (2019, August 5). *Fasted Exercise: Autophagy, Fat Burning and Anti-Aging*. DrJockers.Com. https://drjockers.com/fasted-exercise-autophagy-fat-burning-and-anti-aging/

Jorgenson, A. (2019, June 19). *The Growing Science Behind a Fasting Treatment for Alzheimer's*. Discover Magazine. https://www.discovermagazine.com/health/the-growing-science-behind-a-fasting-treatment-for-alzheimers

Kaushik, S., & Cuervo, A. M. (2012). Chaperone-mediated autophagy: a unique way to enter the lysosome world. *Trends in Cell Biology, 22*(8), 407–417. https://doi.org/10.1016/j.tcb.2012.05.006

Klionsky, D. J., & Codogno, P. (2013). The Mechanism and Physiological Function of Macroautophagy. *Journal of Innate Immunity, 5*(5), 427–433. https://doi.org/10.1159/000351979

Klionsky, D. J., Cregg, J. M., Dunn, W. A., Emr, S. D., Sakai, Y., Sandoval, I. V., Sibirny, A., Subramani, S., Thumm, M., Veenhuis, M., & Ohsumi, Y. (2003). A Unified Nomenclature for Yeast Autophagy-Related Genes. *Developmental Cell, 5*(4), 539–545. https://doi.org/10.1016/s1534-5807(03)00296-x

Kollias, H. (2015, March 25). *Intermittent Fasting for women: Important information you need to know*. Precision Nutrition. https://www.precisionnutrition.com/intermittent-fasting-women

Larkin, A. (2019, July 31). *No, you shouldn't try intermittent fasting while pregnant. Here's why.* Www.Todaysparent.Com. https://www.todaysparent.com/pregnancy/pregnancy-health/intermittent-fasting-while-pregnant/

Levine, B., & Klionsky, D. J. (2017). Autophagy wins the 2016 Nobel Prize in Physiology or Medicine: Breakthroughs in baker's yeast fuel advances in biomedical research. *Proceedings of the National Academy of Sciences of the United States of America, 114*(2), 201–205. https://doi.org/10.1073/pnas.1619876114

Lindberg, S., & Murrell, D. (2018, August 23). *Autophagy: Definition, Diet, Fasting, Cancer, Benefits, and More.* Healthline. https://www.healthline.com/health/autophagy#:~:text=Autophagy%20is%20the%20bo

Masiero, E., Agatea, L., Mammucari, C., Blaauw, B., Loro, E., Komatsu, M., Metzger, D., Reggiani, C., Schiaffino, S., & Sandri, M. (2009). Autophagy Is Required to Maintain Muscle Mass. *Cell Metabolism, 10*(6), 507–515. https://doi.org/10.1016/j.cmet.2009.10.008

Mindfulness Definition | What Is Mindfulness. (2019). Greater Good. https://greatergood.berkeley.edu/topic/mindfulness/definition

Moseley, M. (2020). *Eat, Fast, Live Longer - BBC Horizon 2012 - HD 720p - video dailymotion.* Dailymotion. https://www.dailymotion.com/video/x370lox

Nazish, N. (2020, February 19). *Everything You Need To Know About The Circadian Rhythm Diet.* Forbes. https://www.forbes.com/sites/nomanazish/2020/02/29/everything-you-need-to-know-about-the-circadian-rhythm-diet/#79f1d5fe73f0

Nutrafol Team. (2019, October 11). *Women Need To Know This Before Trying Intermittent Fasting.* Nutrafol. https://nutrafol.com/blog/intermittent-fasting-men-women/

Nutrition, A. (2018, November 6). *The Science Behind Autophagy and Loose Skin.* Accord Nutrition. https://accordnutrition.com/autophagy-loose-skin/

Ohsumi, Y. (2014). Historical landmarks of autophagy research. *Cell Research*, *24*(1), 9–23. https://doi.org/10.1038/cr.2013.169

Oku, M., & Sakai, Y. (2018). Three Distinct Types of Microautophagy Based on Membrane Dynamics and Molecular Machineries. *BioEssays*, *40*(6), 1800008. https://doi.org/10.1002/bies.201800008

Omninutrition. (2019, December 6). *The Story and Benefits of Citrus Bergamot, Autophagy Research*. Www.Ominutrition.Com. https://www.ominutrition.com/the-story-of-citrus-bergamot/#:~:text=Citrus%20bergamot%20is%20a%20truly%20unique%20fruit.&text=%E2%80%9CAutophagy%20is%20about%20recycling%20and

Pathology. (n.d.) *In Merriam-Webster's unabridged dictionary*. https://www.merriam-webster.com/dictionary/pathology#:~:text=1%20%3A%20the%20study%20of%20the,by%20them%20studied%20plant%20pathology

RichieMuscleProdigy. (2011, December 11). *Michael Phelps Workout and Diet*. Muscle Prodigy. https://www.muscleprodigy.com/michael-phelps-workout-and-diet/

Rose, K. (n.d.). *The mental health benefits of fasting*. Www.Amchara.Com. https://www.amchara.com/diet-fasting/the-mental-health-benefits-of-fasting

Salk Institute. (2019, January 24). *Can autophagy stop cancer before it starts?* Healthcare-in-Europe.Com. https://healthcare-in-europe.com/en/news/can-autophagy-stop-cancer-before-it-starts.html

Shah, A. (2020, March 18). *3 Supplements To Take When Intermittent Fasting*. What's Good by V. https://whatsgood.vitaminshoppe.com/supplements-for-intermittent-fasting/

Solon, O. (2017, September 4). The Silicon Valley execs who don't eat for days: "It's not dieting, it's biohacking." *The Guardian*. https://www.theguardian.com/lifeandstyle/2017/sep/04/silicon-valley-ceo-fasting-trend-diet-is-it-safe

Takeshige, K., Baba, M., Tsuboi, S., Noda, T., & Ohsumi, Y. (1992). Autophagy in yeast demonstrated with proteinase-deficient mutants and conditions for its induction. *The Journal of Cell Biology*, *119*(2), 301–311. https://doi.org/10.1083/jcb.119.2.301

Tinsley, G. (2017, December 3). *Does Intermittent Fasting Make You Gain or Lose Muscle?* Healthline. https://www.healthline.com/nutrition/intermittent-fasting-muscle#section3

Uddin, M. S., Stachowiak, A., Mamun, A. A., Tzvetkov, N. T., Takeda, S., Atanasov, A. G., Bergantin, L. B., Abdel-Daim, M. M., & Stankiewicz, A. M. (2018). Autophagy and Alzheimer's Disease: From Molecular Mechanisms to Therapeutic Implications. *Frontiers in Aging Neuroscience*, *10*. https://doi.org/10.3389/fnagi.2018.00004

Whittel, N. (2018, March 6). *Rejuvenate the body with Autophagy tea*. Www.Naomiwhittel.Com. https://www.naomiwhittel.com/rejuvenate-the-body-with-autophagy-tea/

Whittel, N. (2019, December 17). *Avoid Loose Skin When Dieting and Fasting with Autophagy*. Www.Naomiwhittel.Com. https://www.naomiwhittel.com/avoid-loose-skin-with-autophagy/

Winning the Nobel Prize Accelerates Clinical Applications of Autophagy. (2020). http://www.tmd.ac.jp/english/artis-cms/cms-files/Autophagy.pdf

Yu, C. (2020, May 9). *Why Fasting Causes Autophagy — and What's the Deal With That, Anyway?* LIVESTRONG.COM. https://www.livestrong.com/article/13724912-autophagy-fasting/

Images

Figure 1. Pixabay. (2020). Wood [Image]. https://pixabay.com/photos/wood-

Figure 2. Pixabay. (2020). Cells [Image]. https://pixabay.com/illustrations/cellshuman-medical-biology-health-1872666/

Figure 3. Pixabay. (2020). Lemon [Image]. https://pixabay.com/photos/

slice-oflemon-lemon-small-bubbles-2135548/

Figure 4. Pixabay. (2020). Blonde [Image]. https://pixabay.com/photos/

adventure-blonde-hair-exploring-1868817/

Figure 5. Pixabay. (2020). Syringe [Image]. https://pixabay.com/illustrations/

syringe-pill-capsule-morphine-1884784/

Figure 6. Pixabay. (2020). Belly [Image]. https://pixabay.com/photos/

belly-heartlove-girl-relaxation-3186730/

Figure 7. Pixabay. (2020). Girl [Image]. https://pixabay.com/photos/

girl-handsportrait-woman-beauty-3033718/

Figure 8. Pixabay. (2020). Bear [Image]. https://pixabay.com/photos/

teddy-teddy-bearassociation-ill-562960/

Figure 9. Pixabay. (2020). Yoga [Image]. https://pixabay.com/photos/

peoplewoman-yoga-meditation-2573216/

Figure 10. Pixabay. (2020). Berries [Image]. https://pixabay.com/photos/

berriesberry-blackberry-blueberry-1838314/